# HYPNOTHERAPY

# Hypnotherapy

## Cancer, Hospice and Palliative Care

### Carl Anthony

Copyright © 2012 by Carl Anthony.

| Library of Congress Control Number: | | 2012922462 |
|---|---|---|
| ISBN: | Hardcover | 978-1-4797-5489-2 |
| | Softcover | 978-1-4797-5488-5 |
| | Ebook | 978-1-4797-5490-8 |

All rights reserved. No part of this book may be reproduced or transmitted in any form or by any means, electronic or mechanical, including photocopying, recording, or by any information storage and retrieval system, without permission in writing from the copyright owner.

This book was printed in the United States of America.

To order additional copies of this book, contact:
Xlibris Corporation
0-800-644-6988
www.xlibrispublishing.co.uk
Orders@xlibrispublishing.co.uk

# Contents

Acknowledgement .................................................................................. 9

Why write this book? ........................................................................... 11
Hypnotherapy: A Brief History of Hypnosis ...................................... 25
What is Hypnosis ................................................................................. 31
'The Dying Process—The Transition From Life to Death' ............... 38
How can hypnotherapy help with cancer? ......................................... 50
Relaxation ............................................................................................. 56
Dying Regrets ....................................................................................... 60
The Dying Process: The Transition From Life to Death .................. 65
Loss of a Loved One ........................................................................... 70
Living With Cancer: Relaxation for Chemotherapy ......................... 75
Relaxation for Brain Tumour .............................................................. 79
Pre-Surgery .......................................................................................... 82
Living With Cancer: Relaxation ......................................................... 86
Hypnosis and the Relief of Pain ......................................................... 91
Writing Your Own Hypnosis Scripts ............................................... 104
Strength and Courage ....................................................................... 170

Index .................................................................................................. 181

This book is written in the honour of my late father Albert James Gathern, who passed away of lung cancer in 1991

You are my shining light

Until we meet again one day . . .

# Acknowledgement

Great thanks for the many people, whom I have met over the years, with whose help this book has been written. Their support, learning, and teaching have enabled me to realise and work with the words 'I am that I am'. My destiny is indeed in my very own hands.

A special thank you to Claire, Eileen, and my soon-to-be wife, Sarah

Thank you and with much love

Carl

# Why write this book?

My name is Carl Anthony, and I am a professionally trained hypnotherapist and shamanic practitioner. I am also currently studying a two-year advanced diploma in psychotherapeutic counselling, and the reason for writing this book is very simple. I believe hypnotherapy has a very important role to play in the welfare of each and every one of us. How we relate to others is how we relate to ourselves, and through the practice of hypnosis, we can become the person we were born to be. This includes the practice of hypnotherapy during our years as we grow spiritually and also as we end our lives during the transition into the afterlife.

During my practice as a hypnotherapist and a counsellor, I have worked with many people with many issues concerning the stigma of death. It is very evident from working with support groups and in my private practice that there is a need for an understanding of both the patients' needs as well as the care and understanding of the carers. This doesn't mean just the wonderful job that all nurses and doctors do but also what it is like for the close relatives and friends, who are quite often overlooked at the time when they need help themselves.

Hypnotherapy has a role to play, and I write this book so that others too may benefit from the peace that hypnotherapy brings to so many, many people. It has to be said at this point that I am not saying that hypnotherapy is a cure for cancer; rather, that by using this tool, hypnotherapy can work alongside the conventional medical methods used with such cancer patients, thus helping in the overall welfare of the patient and carer alike.

The idea of doing this came simply while I was doing my hypnotherapy training, where part of the course covered the subject of hypnotherapy and ways that it could help people with medical conditions. My father died twenty years ago from lung cancer; he deteriorated and died before my own eyes. It was my first experience of seeing a person die. I felt there was nothing I could do for him. It was a long and painful death, and, at that time, there were no alternative ways of dealing with his condition and no support groups to help ease the pain, grief, and loss of himself, close relatives, and friends.

The following is an extract from the essay I had written; the seeds had been sown, and for me, there was no looking back:

'There is plenty of evidence to suggest that Hypnotherapy can help people with cancer, even if it is only to improve their quality of life for the time being. The reason why Hypnotherapy can be relevant is because mind, body and spirit are all interconnected and any treatment needs to take this into account. The extraordinary advances in medical science have been due to a greater understanding of how the body works and this has led to an emphasis on physical treatment (radiotherapy, chemotherapy etc), but the mind has its part to play as well.

Hypnotherapy can therefore be used alongside the conventional medical treatments for cancer, and for a number of different purposes, as the following list shows:

## 1. Relaxation versus stress

It is generally accepted that stress can reduce the effectiveness of the human immune system, so changing the body's ability to deal with cancer cells. Finding out that you have cancer is certainly stressful and, if you were not stressed before, you probably will be when you receive the diagnosis. Stress is an attitude of mind, you cannot control the external world but you can decide how you are going to react to it.

There are a number of ways of improving relaxation, and hypnotherapy is a very effective one. When you first have hypnotherapy you will be taken through a progressive relaxation, relaxing the body and then the mind. Of course it is not enough to be relaxed only when you are with your hypnotherapist, it is essential (where possible) to teach your subject how to do self-hypnosis, giving them a simple but very effective technique for taking themselves into a relaxing hypnotic trance. After a little practice your subject will find that they can reduce their feelings of stress and feel much better as a result.

## 2. Psychoneuroimmunology

The relatively new study of psychoneuroimmunology has shown that there is a relationship between the mind and the human immune system. Encouraging the client to think about their immune system, and focus on what it can do for them, does have a beneficial effect.

Hypnotherapy will begin with guided visualisation of the immune system and will ask the client to give themselves affirmations about their immune system while they are in self-hypnosis, which they will be asked to do at least once a day (or done for them if they are not able to) The subject may also be asked to do drawings showing themselves, the cancer, their immune system and their treatment. They will be encouraged to think about their immune system, together with their treatment, as being strong and powerful with the cancer cells.

## 3. Side-effects

There are a number of side-effects to cancer treatment which can be distressing or uncomfortable. It may be possible to eliminate or reduce these side-effects using hypnotherapy. For example, anticipatory nausea may arise in people going for chemotherapy. The fact that it happens before rather than after the treatment indicates that it has a psychological cause (although it is nonetheless nausea).

People taking tamoxifen sometimes experience hot flushes. We know that blushing has a psychological cause, and can be treated using hypnotherapy, so we can use similar techniques to help reduce hot flushes. Other side-effects such as fear of dying or depression can also be helped with hypnotherapy.

## 4 Preparation for surgery

Hypnosis can be used in place or alongside of a general anaesthetic for some forms of surgery. This is of particular interest for those who find the after effects of a general anaesthetic to be unpleasant.

However it is more common to use hypnotherapy to help prepare for surgery. This takes several forms:

- Firstly, a relaxed subject who is expecting the operation to go well and who is expecting to recover quickly is likely to make better progress than one who is fearful or anxious.
- Secondly, the subject can be trained to respond to suggestions given by the surgeon during an operation. While under a general anaesthetic a person's conscious mind may be closed but their sense of hearing and their unconscious mind are still open. The surgeon can therefore give suggestions about blood flow and healing, to which the person's unconscious mind can respond.

## 5. Self—confidence and empowerment

When a person is told that they have cancer there is a natural tendency for this to dominate their thinking and for them not to be able to see beyond their recovery, and because they are in a situation which they may not have had to face before, they may feel over-reliant on others (doctors, consultant, nursing staff) and feel they have lost control of their own lives.

Hypnotherapy can help to re-establish their self-confidence, empower them in their dealings with others, and extend their focus to what they want to do with the rest of their lives. They will be encouraged to think about their goals (in addition to possible recovery), and to consider these goals when in self-hypnosis. Establishing a goal as important in the unconscious mind will result in much better motivation.

## 6. Other issues

People with cancer have the same issues as everybody else, but the cancer may bring a particular issue to the fore. For example a needle phobia which may have been largely irrelevant in the past, may become very significant for somebody who is now visiting hospital much more than before.

Emotional issues which have been put to one side in the past may become more important for somebody considering a reduced life expectancy, and hypnotherapy can help with this. Emotional issues can arise both from the practical and personal level. For example:

## Practical

- Changes in the environment due to changes in mobility
- Changes in modes of transport (if people have to stop driving)
- Changes in ability to perform the tasks of daily living
- Changes in financial position
- Changes in input from external sources (dealing with the medical profession, benefit agencies etc)
- Changes to employment or career
- Possible loss of available time (through loss of mobility or fatigue)

## Personal

- Ability to carry out day-to-day care
- Ability to perform tasks or go out alone
- Acceptance of care needs
- Possible stigmas of some conditions
- Effects on intimate relationships
- Role reversal within the family unit
- Change in the way the person sees themselves in relationship to others in the workplace and within the family
- Change in goals and dreams

From this many emotional feelings can be associated with those changes, and hypnotherapy can help with this, for example:

- Loss and associated grief
- Anger
- Insecurity
- Loss of independence/increase on dependence on others
- Depression
- Negativity about the future
- Denial
- Hopelessness
- Feelings of being a burden
- Feelings of being a failure
- Anxiety
- Fear
- Dealing with the emotion or hidden emotion of others

- Not understanding why
- Changes in the way the person experiences feelings
- Low self-esteem
- Lack of previous confidence
- Changes in identity
- Confusion
- Worthlessness
- Obsesssion over the illness
- Isolation
- Fear of dying

Not all people will experience all of the above during their illness and the list is not exhaustive.

## 7. Carers

A person caring for somebody they love, and having to face the fact that they may die, will certainly benefit from the relaxation techniques and process, providing an understanding that hypnotherapy can provide. A carer may need help to focus on their own needs, as well as those of the person they are caring for.

Hypnotherapy can also provide respite for carers in a professional setting, helping them to come to terms with their own emotional problems surrounding their care work.'

I think it is very important that anybody who wishes to work with cancer patients gets written permission from their doctor or consultant (where possible) before they embark on any form of hypnotherapy.

In this part of the book, I feel it is a relevant time to discuss the fact that not only is it important to get permission from the relevant person, but it is also important to have a sound understanding of cancer and the process before embarking on any hypnotherapy treatment. This, I feel, is ethical to the needs of the patient, carer, and family alike.

Dying is a part of life, and we should respect ourselves and others, not only in our years as we grow but also in the years as we prepare to die. We should respect and honour other peoples' wishes as if they were our own, and in turn, we will earn respect in all that we do at such a critical time in peoples' life.

## Who gets cancer?

- Each year, nearly three hundred thousand people are diagnosed with cancer in the United Kingdom.
- It has been estimated that more than one in three people will develop cancer at some point in their lifetime.

Cancers can occur at any age, but the risk of developing cancer does increase with age.

- Three-quarters of all newly diagnosed cancers occur in people aged sixty or over.
- Less than one in a hundred of cancers are diagnosed in children, aged fourteen or under.
- About one in ten of cancers are diagnosed in people aged twenty-five to forty-nine.

Some cancers are very common and some are very rare. For men, the most common is prostate cancer (24 per cent), followed by lung cancer (15 per cent), colon and rectal cancer (14 per cent), and bladder cancer (5 per cent).

For women, the most common is breast cancer (31 per cent), colon and rectal cancer (12 per cent), lung cancer, (12 per cent), and womb cancer (5 per cent).

Nearly a third of all cancers diagnosed in children are leukaemia. Teenagers and young people are more likely to be diagnosed with Hodgkin lymphoma, testicular cancer, melanoma, and leukaemia.

The most common types of cancer in adults aged twenty-five to forty-nine are breast cancer, melanoma, and bowel and cervical cancer.

- There are over two hundred types of cancer; although the cause of some of these is not known, we do know some of the risk factors that can increase a person's risk of developing cancer. Increasing with age is a risk factor that we can't do anything about, but we can make lifestyle choices about some of the other risk factors such as stopping smoking, eating a balanced diet, cutting down on alcohol, and getting regular exercises. Hypnotherapy can play a vital role in this, as well as reducing the stress, anxiety, and worry that can occur during these times.

We are getting better at recognising and treating cancer, so today, many people can be cured. Even if cancer can't be cured, it can often be controlled with treatment for months or years.

## Signs and symptoms

Cancer can often be managed more easily when it is diagnosed in the early stages, being aware of your body and what is normal for you, and reporting symptoms to your GP can help to make sure that if you do have cancer, it is diagnosed as early as possible.

There are some common signs and symptoms that may alert you to the fact that something is new or different. A doctor should be contacted if you have any of the following:

- A lump
- Cough, breathlessness, or hoarseness that doesn't go away
- Changes in bowel habit
- Abnormal bleeding
- Changes in a mole
- Unexplained weight loss
- Bleeding

## Types of cancer

It is important to know what type of cancer one has because different types of cancer can behave very differently and respond to different treatments.

Cancers are grouped in two ways, according to the following:
Site: the part of the body where the cancer first developed
Cell type: the type of cell the cancer started from

The most common *sites* in which cancer develops include the following:

- Skin
- Lungs
- Breasts
- Prostate
- Colon and rectum

Our body is made up of millions of cells. The cells organised together make up all of our tissues and organs. There are different types of cells to carry out different functions in the body.

The main types of cells in our body are as follows:

- Epithelial cells. These cover the outside of the body (as skin) and make up tissues that line the inside of our bodies and cover our organs.
- Cells of the blood and lymphatic system. These are found in our blood, in the bone marrow (where blood cells are made), and in the lymphatic system (which fights infection).
- Connective tissue cells. These cells are found in supportive and connective tissues in our body, such as the muscles, bones, and fatty tissue.

Cancers that start in each of these types of cells have different names. They are as follows:

# Carcinomas

Cancers that start in epithelial cells are called carcinomas. They are the most common types of cancer in adults and make up 80 to 90 per cent out of every cancers. Most lung, breast, prostate, and bowel cancers are carcinomas.

There are different types of epithelial cells. They are as follows:

- Squamous cells are found in the skin and cover the surface of many parts of the body, including the mouth, gullet (oesophagus), and the airways.
- Adenocarcinoma cells form the lining of all the glands in the body, including those in the breasts, bowel, stomach, ovaries, and prostate.
- Urothelial (transitional) cells line the bladder and parts of the urinary system.
- Basal cells are found in the skin.

Carcinomas may start in any of these types of cells.

## Leukaemia and lymphomas

Cancers that start in the blood or the bone marrow (the tissues where blood cells are formed to fight infection in the body) are called leukaemia.

Cancers that start in the lymphatic system (which helps the body fight infection) are called lymphomas.

Leukaemia and lymphomas are quite rare, making up fewer than 7 per cent of cancers.

## Sarcomas

Cancers that start in connective tissue cells are called sarcomas.

- Sarcomas are quite rare.
- They make up fewer than 1 per cent of all cancers.

Sarcomas are split into two main types. They are as follows:

- Bone sarcomas, which are found in the bones
- Soft-tissue sarcomas, which develop in the other supportive tissues of the body

Cancers can develop in other types of cells, but these cancers are rare. Brain cancers are the most common cancers in this group.

## How is cancer treated?

There are different types of cancer treatment.

Some are used to treat cancer in a particular (local) area of the body. These are called local treatments. They include surgery and radiotherapy. Other treatments can treat cancer in more than one part of the body at a time. These are called systemic treatments. Chemotherapy, hormonal therapy, and biological therapy generally work in this way.

The main types of treatment of cancer are listed below; it is quite common for a combination of treatments to be used:

- Surgery
- Radiotherapy
- Chemotherapy
- Hormonal therapy
- Biological therapy

When writing this book, I had to ask myself some strong questions. I work to a very strict code of conduct and ethics, and, ultimately, I work for the clients and their highest good in the best possible way available for me at that time. One particular question did give me some very good food for thought, though, and is very relevant for the writing of this book.

Should hypnotherapy only be practiced by medically trained therapists?

This is a very good question, and I myself do have to answer that question with a definite and resounding 'yes'!

This question is not a new topic of conversation, and many people do have their own values, opinions, and ideas on this.

The following is taken from various other professional therapists, and I do agree with them.

'Should the same be said for acupuncturists, radiologists, podiatrists etc? I think that there is absolutely no reason why properly trained clinical hypnotherapists should not treat suitable patients. All that needs done is that the training and regulatory bodies train to s standard that is approved by the medical establishment.'

'A problem is that clinically trained hypnotherapists are so effective that it may tread on the toes of the medical profession who will then wish to control it.'

'I would go so far as to say, that most illness is a physical manifestation of a disturbance-how shall I describe it without sounding all new age—deeper energies that we have trapped in the body by our inside out way of experiencing life. Its of importance to take into account those subtle energies manifest into all kinds of disease!'

'The way I see it is that maybe medics need to be trained in the understanding of mind-body energy before they are allowed to practice hypnotherapy.'

'Most hypnotherapists have years of training and personal and professional development.'

The following extract from a professional registered nurse sums up for me what it is that hypnotherapy can do to help with the dying process and the transition from life to death. If one person, *just one* person, can be of benefit from the role hypnotherapy can play in cancer, hospice, and palliative care, then the many, many hours writing and researching this book would have been worth it.

'The Dying Process or the Transition From Life to Death has been observed by me personally.' For thirty-four years of my life, I have been in the Nursing Profession, and if I should add to that my years of being a nursing assistant that would make it forty years of nurturing and helping people. Yes, there is a need to add on those nursing assistant years here, because in them contains the witness to the most horrific death I have ever seen!

As a nursing assistant, it was my job to come in and do vital signs. At that time we used glass thermometers. I had already taken them out of the cleaning solution, and shaken them all down, of course keeping the red tips separated from the blue tips.(Smile Nurses!) Entering this patients room, he was very hot and sweaty and moaning and groaning and thrashing about. I turned him over, finding him very hot, and red as a lobster! Just standing near him made me very warm. I could not believe my eyes when I took the thermometer out! His temperature was off the end of the thermometer. I reported it and retook it with the same result . . . This man died the most miserable death, I have ever seen! I felt like he was being tortured, and I all of seventeen years old slept with the lights on for a very long time.

And then compare to the sweetest departure from this world that I have seen. Sweet lady, and I was feeding her, dinner. She only wanted the ice cream! Imagine my horror when after the second spoon of ice cream, her eyes rolled back up in her head and she died, right there in front of me! I ran screaming for the nurses, who came in the room and did CPR on her unsuccessfully. I cried, and was only consolable when one of the nurses told me this, 'You gave her, her last taste of sweetness before she left this world!'

I have come to discover that the period before death can be difficult as the body is shutting down or being consumed by disease. During this time, it's easy for the mind to become overwhelmed and unable to manage. And now being a Professional nurse; know that during that time the body is in what we call Multisystem Organ Failure. A variety of symptoms manifest at this time. In the hospital settings, we do many things to help with them.

My mom decided she would die at home. When I arrived there, the 'Angel Nurses', my name for Hospice Nurses were on the case. Wonderful, but when I saw my mom, not in as bad a shape as the man described above, but almost in my mind. But some many years later now and a Registered Nurse, I knew she was in the multi organ system failure part of death at this time. As I said, I had seen this before!

But this time, and having just learned Hypnotherapy, I wasn't going to stand by and hear her (mom) moan like this. So I went to the car and read frantically over my newly learned Hypnotherapy scripts, returned to her bedside, paced her breathing, slowed hers down, and counted her down and led her in a meditation of Psalms twenty three and to the Table to have a talk with Jesus, and I just said to tell him all about it and talk with Him . . . and during that time, I sang, 'I come to the Garden Alone' while the dew is still on the roses . . . All the while watching her and I knew when she had reached that table to talk with Him as such a peace came over her body, (I can't even begin to imagine that divine moment and talk with Jesus) and then she scared me! I was so enjoying that peace that had come over her when her eyes opened and she spoke with peace. She died peacefully over the next day.

What I learned from all of my experiences of seeing and watching people as they transition over, is this is a time for friends and family to step in and help. Anything we can do to reduce worry and create an uplifting atmosphere will help make for an easier time for your loved one while passing. I so understand that some will be able to do something and understand and some won't, I personally have some family members who to this day do not understand how my mom's strength returned for that short period of time before she passed on.

Even so, anything you can do to help a person at this time, please do. Hold their hand, rub their forehead, sing, pray or do whatever you do in your tradition. But please know that, as the body is going through the shutting down process of death, that person is going through so much.

Nursing taught me that hearing is the last sense to leave the body. 'So be careful what you say and do, do respect the body of that person, preserve their dignity, even then!'

I have to say that after reading stories like that, even though I believe hypnotherapy should only be done after the relevant proper training, there must be *an exception to the rule*. How can anyone be denied help at such a time as this when they are in the dying process and in the transition from life to death?

If you are able and willing, then you must do whatever it is you can to help in the dying process or the transition from life to death.

# Hypnotherapy:
# A Brief History of Hypnosis

A detailed history of hypnosis and its uses through the ages would be very lengthy, as it is one of the oldest therapies known and used by man. I have opted for a brief history as there are so many other good books and points of reference out there on the subject for the reader to explore if he or she so wishes.

Its origins go back many, many millennia, and, indeed, many ancient cultures and civilisations from the Ancient Egyptians, Greeks, Romans, Indians, Chinese, Persians, and Sumerians show extensive studies in hypnosis, altered states of consciousness, and parapsychology. Hypnosis was considered as a cure for many physical and emotional ailments and disorders.

In other words, hypnosis is at least more than six thousand years old, and some scholars claim that it could be as old as prehistory, as certain cave paintings show priests that are apparently in a state of trance as well as geometrical designs thought to depict visions seen in an altered level of consciousness.

Although there was some use of hypnosis by the Druids in Ancient Britain and Gaul, the development and introduction of hypnosis to the modern world is attributable to Islamic scientists of the Middle Ages.

Between the ninth and fourteenth centuries, there was a great flowering of civilisation in the Mediterranean and Middle East which laid the foundations of modern science as we know it; medical and philosophical knowledge from Ancient Greece, Egypt, and early Eastern civilisations was revitalised.

During that revival, a deep understanding of human psychology was achieved, and therapeutic processes such as analysis, altered states of consciousness, and hypnosis were used to alleviate emotional distress and sufferings, thus preceding psychotherapy and hypnotherapy as we know them today by quite a few centuries.

From the fifteenth and sixteenth centuries onwards, physicians from many nations developed further and refined the concept of hypnosis and its uses. Even though this knowledge spread throughout the European continent and to the British Isles, it remained mostly confined to scientists, physicians, and universities and never quite reached the attention of the less-educated people.

It was 'reintroduced' to the West in the eighteenth century when Western explorers got in contact with the practice of hypnotism in the Middle East and the Far East.

In the eighteenth century, the most influential figure in the development of hypnosis was Dr Frantz Anton Mesmer (1734-1815), an Austrian physician who was a charismatic and, at times, controversial personality.

He used magnets and metal frames to perform 'passes' over the patient to remove 'blockages' (i.e., the causes of diseases) in the magnetic forces in the body—nowadays, we call such forces 'life energy'—and to induce a trance-like state. He soon discovered that he could reach equally successful results by passing his hands over the patient, which he did for many hours at times.

Mesmer named this method 'animal magnetism' and worked in Austria, Switzerland, and Germany before he settled down in practice in France. Although he achieved many successes, he was soon derided and ostracised by the medical community, and it is generally thought that his healing sessions held in front of the public and medical profession were such theatrical performances that the excessive showmanship he displayed led to his work being ridiculed and his tangible results scorned at.

Another contributing factor that was to his discredit is believed to be the jealousy afforded to him from his medical colleagues, along with the unorthodox methods to achieve results. He believed he could store his 'animal magnetism' in baths of iron filings and transfer it to his patients with rods or by 'mesmeric passes'!

However, his name survived the passing of time and was immortalised in our vocabulary by the verb 'mesmerise', which means to hold someone's attention to the exclusion of anything else so as to create a trance-like state, which, in other words, was to hypnotise that person. Not only his name survived in our vocabulary, but also his method, which was named mesmerism.

After Mesmer's death, one of his disciples, Amand de Puysegur, carried on his work and took it one step further. He discovered that the spoken word and direct commands induced trance easily and noticeably faster than 'mesmeric passes' and that a person could be operated upon without pain and anaesthesia when in trance. This technique was used for many following decades by surgeons in France: Dr Recamier, who performed the first recorded operation without anaesthesia in 1821 and in England with Dr Ellotson and Dr Parker (nicknamed Painless Parker!)

However, the record for surgery under trance belongs to Dr James Esdaile, an English physician, who performed his first operation without anaesthetic in India and reached an incredible tally of three hundred major operations and a thousand minor operations, using hypnosis or mesmerism as it was called at that time.

Soon after, chloroform was discovered and mesmerism dropped out of favour as an anaesthetic; it was much faster to inject a patient than induce a state of trance!

The next impulse in the history of hypnosis was given by the Scottish optometrist, Dr James Braid, who discovered by accident that a person fixating an object could easily reach a trance-like state without the help of the mesmeric passes advocated by Dr Mesmer.

In 1841, he published his findings, refuted Mesmer's work, and inaccurately named his discovery 'hypnotism' based on the Greek word 'hypnos' which means 'sleep'; it was a total misnomer, as hypnosis is certainly not *sleep*; yet the name remained, and mesmerism became hypnotism.

Another page was turned in the history of hypnosis and by the mid-1800s, two schools of hypnosis were created in France, one by Dr Jean-Martin Charcot, in Paris, and the other in Nancy by Dr Benheim and Dr Liebault.

Further progresses were made in refining the concept of hypnosis; however, it was not without heated debates and arguments!

Dr Charcot stated that hypnosis could only be the result of physical or neurological stimulation, while the Nancy school's view was that hypnosis is a natural state available to everyone using free will.

Present days' use of hypnosis follows the latter belief!

Some twenty years later, in 1891, the British Medical Association drafted a resolution in favour of the use of hypnosis in medicine, but it was not approved until 1955, sixty-four years later!

Another precursor of modern hypnosis and self-development was Dr Emile Coue who, at the end of the nineteenth century, was a believer in autosuggestion and in the role of the hypnotist as a facilitator of changes and healing in the client's condition by involving the total participation of the client in the hypnosis process.

His well-known self-help statement 'Day by day in every way I am getting better and better' is still used in most self-improvement therapies.

Around the same period, Sigmund Freud, the father of psychoanalysis, used hypnosis in his early work but soon became disillusioned by the concept. It is believed he did not have the patience necessary for hypnosis and was not a good hypnotist!

As we know, he focused his attention on analysis and free association. In many ways, his 'defection' was damaging to hypnosis, particularly in the context of psychology, as it created enduring prejudices and misconceptions which have only started to fade in recent times.

With the development of psychoanalysis and the use of anaesthetics, the interest in hypnosis somewhat declined; however, in the beginning of the twentieth century, Russian scientists worked on the concept and mechanisms of hypnosis.

The most illustrious one, Ivan P. Pavlov, is best known for his discovery of the conditional reflex, in spite of the fact he was awarded a Nobel Prize in 1904 for his work on digestion!

After First World War, hypnosis and its therapeutic uses experienced a revival when psychiatrists realised that soldiers suffering traumas (paralysis and amnesia) of a psychological rather than physical origin were responding well to hypnosis and were rapidly cured.

Despite this renewed interest, European scientists who had previously been to the forefront of the hypnosis saga for centuries devoted much less time and energy to the subject, possibly by becoming more accepted, and less controversial hypnosis was attracting less passion.

Although hypnosis was officially approved as a tool in medicine by the British Medical Association in 1955, most of the furthering in therapeutic hypnosis in the twentieth century took place in the United States. In 1958, only three years after the BMA, the American Medical Association recognised the therapeutic use of hypnosis.

There are many therapists, researchers, and scientists—far too many for the scope of this book—who have made significant contributions to hypnosis. It is widely believed that in the twentieth century, the two main figures in the field were Milton H. Erickson and Dr William J Bryan.

M. H. Erickson was a psychotherapist who made intensive use of hypnosis in his work. He was a great and fast observer of people and could rapidly build rapport with his clients. Metaphors, imagery, confusing statements, surprise, and humour were part of his arsenal of therapeutic tools. His hypnotic methods, nowadays called 'ericksonian hypnosis', have, without a doubt, added another dimension to modern hypnotherapy.

William J. Bryan Jr was the first full-time US medical practitioner of hypnosis and created the American Institute of Hypnosis.

In the 1970s, a discovery was made in the field of self-improvement and the harnessing of inner resources. Although it is not directly related to hypnosis, many of its techniques can be used with hypnosis or as an aid to hypnotic therapy.

It is a simple but brilliant technique created by Richard Brandler, an information scientist, and John Grindler, a linguistic professor; they named it NLP (neurolinguistic programming).

It came about, in large part, by its two founders studying, understanding, and developing methods used by Milton H. Erickson in psychotherapy. NLP is a tool for improvement, using our neurology and thinking patterns (neuro), our way of expressing our thoughts and their influence on us (linguistic), and our patterns of behaviour and goals setting (programming). It has been described as the ultimate software for the brain.

In the last three to four decades of the last century, we have witnessed an abundance of self-help and positive-thinking therapies and methods, some of them openly using hypnosis, others more covertly, technological advancements, such as TV, and the globalisation of information through the Internet, have also made use of the various uses of hypnosis.

The benefits of hypnotherapy are more and more recognised and for those who search for betterment of themselves and of their lives, both during and towards the end.

*Hypnotherapy* is *available* and *very effective.*

# What is Hypnosis

Definitions of hypnosis are aplenty!

Practically, everyone, hypnosis professional or not, will give a different answer to the question. Basically, hypnosis is a state of trance induced by suggestions, and being in trance is really a very natural thing; in fact, we all do it at some point in our life every day (although we may never realise it at the time!). We could, for example, be engrossed in a book or a film and our attention is totally focused on what we are seeing or reading; it becomes our reality, and the real world around us does not 'exist' any more.

Daydreaming is another type of trance which occurs naturally and automatically when our body and mind are in need of rest after a time of alertness; long-distance driving or driving along the same route every day creates a trance-like state, during which you use your driving skills competently but at the end of your journey, you have little or no recall of it. This is because everything that you have learned is stored in your subconscious.

For example, because you have already learned to drive, your driving skill is stored in your subconscious. As you begin your journey, you get in your car, you manoeuvre on to the road, move on to a continuous flow of traffic, and reach a consistent speed. Now your conscious mind is free. That is, because the knowledge required for driving exists in your subconscious, your conscious mind drifts off, allowing your subconscious to become more active. You may become so engrossed in your thoughts that you drive in the direction of your office when your actual destination is the shops or the cinema! When your attention is needed to change lanes, avoid something in the road, stop at the junction, or slow down for lights, your conscious mind comes into play again.

You may even arrive at your destination and wonder how you got there so quickly (you may even wonder how you got you to this page in this book!).

Driving is only one automatic activity. Whenever you do anything automatic, your conscious mind is diverted from your subconscious and you are more likely to go into an hypnotic state, such as the one described in the car.

These are examples of trance-like states we experience spontaneously, as opposed to trances used in hypnotherapy as well as in yoga, meditation, and creative visualisation which are induced deliberately by a therapist or by one's self (self-hypnosis).

Within science, there is no debate as to whether hypnosis exists or even works. Science simply cannot agree on what it is and how it works, although as the British Society of Clinical and Experimental Hypnosis states as follows:

'In therapy, hypnosis usually involves the person experiencing a sense of deep relaxation with their attention narrowed down, and focused on appropriate suggestions made by the therapist.'

These suggestions help people make positive changes within themselves, and in a hypnotherapy session, you are always in control, and you are not made to do anything that you wouldn't normally do.

It is generally accepted that all hypnosis is ultimately self-hypnosis, and a hypnotherapist merely helps to facilitate your experience—hypnotherapy is not, in fact, about being made to do things; it is the opposite; it is about self-empowerment. Hypnotherapy is a great tool that can help you change and grow and to help you realise your full potential, ultimately being able to do what it is 'you' want to do and not what someone 'else' wants you to do!

*Whatever stage of your life you are in, hypnotherapy can help you.*

Contrary to popular belief, hypnosis is not a state of deep sleep. It does involve the induction of a trance-like condition, but when in it, the patient is actually in an enhanced state of awareness, concentrating on the hypnotist's voice. In this state, the conscious mind is suppressed and the subconscious mind is revealed.

The therapist is able to suggest ideas, concepts, and lifestyle adaptations to the patient, the seeds of which become firmly planted and the practice of promoting healing or positive development in any such way is known as hypnotherapy, and as such, hypnotherapy is a kind of psychotherapy.

Hypnotherapy aims to reprogramme patterns of behaviour within the mind, enabling irrational fears, phobias, negative thoughts, and suppressed emotions to be overcome. As the body is released from conscious control during the relaxed trance-like state of hypnosis, breathing becomes slower and deeper, the pulse rate drops, and the metabolic rate falls.

Similar changes along nervous pathways and hormonal channels enable the sensation of pain to become less acute and the awareness of unpleasant symptoms, such as nausea or indigestion, to be alleviated.

Hypnosis is thought to work by altering our state of consciousness, and we have a conscious mind and an unconscious mind, which work together and communicate with each other at all times.

The conscious mind is rational, logical, and functions on facts; it is the mind involved in our everyday thinking. The subconscious mind is creative, imaginative, and irrational; it also has a huge 'memory bank' where every event in our lives and emotions associated to it are filed. It works by association linking a present situation to a past event without using logic. Our subconscious mind is the seat of our own individual programming beliefs, ideas, emotions, thoughts, and behaviours. In addition, the subconscious mind controls the main functions of the body (breathing, blood circulation, digestion, elimination, tissue regeneration, hormonal production, etc . . . .); it keeps us alive.

Hypnosis is an altered state of consciousness which involves relaxation, concentration, goal orientation, and suggestibility. It allows the mind to easily and deeply focus on one subject, and furthermore, it is the only time we can communicate with the subconscious mind and reprogramme it.

During hypnosis, the conscious and subconscious minds receive the same message given through suggestions, but the conscious mind records it logically, while the subconscious mind absorbs it by association (sometimes called free association).

Let us take the example of someone who suffers from a phobia of spiders; consciously, the person knows that it is a small creature, unable to harm a human being (in our temperature climate), and can easily recognise that fearing such a small creature is irrational; however, all this logical approach does not remove the end result: *fear*. Why does this happen? The answer is the programming in the person's subconscious mind: spiders are equal to danger, often caused by a past frightening experience during childhood or 'inherited' from phobic parents, siblings, or friends.

Hypnotic suggestions given in such a case will state, for example, that a spider is a small and harmless creature and that when in contact with an arachnid, the person will remain calm, unconcerned, and free from fear. The conscious mind will receive the message logically—small, harmless, and, therefore, not dangerous—while the subconscious mind will accept by 'free association' that seeing a spider is *now* a non-threatening situation.

Sometimes the suggestions have to be repeated again and again to be able to alter the subconscious programming from its original position of 'spiders are equal to danger' to a new position of 'spiders are not equal to harm'.

As we look more closely at the hypnotic state, the development of science has enabled us to measure the electrical activity of the brain. The method involved is called electroencephalography (EEG) and measures the electrical activity of the brain known as brain waves.

There are four main types of brain wave, each varying in frequency, and are all associated with each of our levels of consciousness. They are as follows:

## Beta waves (fifteen to forty cycles per second)

These are characteristic of an engaged, alert, and focused mind. A person engaging in active conversation and normal reflective and motor response would be in beta rhythm, while those engaging in teaching, debating, and so on, would be in the higher ranges of beta waves.

The level of consciousness would be alert and, in the present moment, something we are all doing on a daily basis.

## Alpha waves (nine to fourteen cycles per second)

These are slower than the beta waves and represent a less-aroused state. There is a relaxation of the body, slowed breathing and pulse, and a withdrawal into one's self. There is also a direction of attention to imagined activity, dialogue, and times of creativity. This is a light trance of hypnosis and guided meditation. As we relax more, we enter into a deeper state as the waves slow down.

The level of consciousness would be one of daydreaming and light trance.

## Theta waves (four to eight cycles per second)

These are associated with dreaming and some meditative states; they are present when there is serene calmness, medium to deep hypnosis, and an emotional surge. Theta waves are associated with our subconscious mind where we hold all our past experiences—thoughts and behaviour patterns.

Activation of theta waves sometimes bring up suppressed memories, bringing them to the notice of the conscious mind, which may be emotionally painful but may also, with the correct support, be healing. Here is where we access our intuition and our gateway to learning.

In the theta state, there will be a loss of awareness of one's surroundings. Eyes will be closed with an increased awareness of internal functions such as heartbeat or breathing. There will also be an increased receptivity of the senses, and there will be an intensified range of imagery.

Level of consciousness would be a medium or deep trance.

In the theta wave condition, there is a close region between a medium trance and a deep trance. Depending on the level of trance, you can move between the two but still be in the theta wave range.

During a deep trance, there will be a further reduction of activity and energy output; there will be a limpness or stiffness of the limbs and a narrowing of attention span.

There will also be increased suggestibility, along with an illusion of the senses. There will be a loss of auditory receptivity and environmental awareness with a heightened function of the creative process.

## Delta waves (one to four cycles per second)

These are produced in our subconscious mind and when we are in our slowest deepest state of rest and there are no other waves active. This is a state of detached awareness and sleep, possibly representative of very deep hypnosis.

The waves never go down to zero, and a dreamless sleep will take you down to the lowest frequency of two or three cycles per second. There will be a suspension of voluntary exercise and a severe reduction or absence of conscious thoughts.

The level of consciousness would be sleep.

When working with hypnosis, you will need to be working in the alpha and theta wave brain states, which is where behaviour modification will occur. During these states, you will be most susceptible to post-hypnotic suggestions. It is important to remember and understand that no two individuals will have identical experiences, as they progress from the state of alertness to the deep trance. You may be far more suggestible in a moderate trance than someone else in a deep trance. It is even possible for someone in a light trance to accept a major suggestion, such as numbness of a body part.

But generally speaking, when you are in a trance state in which you are receptive to hypnotic suggestion, you will be likely to experience relaxation, sleepiness, a rigidity or limpness in the muscles of your arms and legs, skin warmth or coldness, sensations of tingling or feelings of electricity, and narrowness of attention.

It is also common to have a sense of strangeness or unreality. This means that you may see yourself or your surroundings in a new way, more detached or more connected than usual.

One subject described his feelings as 'I felt as if my mind were floating above my physical body'. Another said, 'My entire body felt as if it were made of warm material, that I could bend into shape and mould around my body.' Further said, 'The windows of the room seemed to squint shut like eyes, and then I was in a very comfortable darkness.'

Some subjects will not have any sensations similar to these, and the way each person responds to hypnosis depends upon his attitudes, preconceived ideas, expectations, and sometimes even fantasies.

To summarise, our brains work with us in the following ways:

- If we give our brain a suggestion, it will follow.
- Our brains will externalise the instructions that it has internally—what we say will be a representation of their internal world.
- Brains leave and return to the present moment, allowing daydreaming and creativity.
- Brains create our mental state.
- Brains do not stop—they go forwards and backwards and around an issue—both positive and negative thought spirals.
- Brains make sense of experience.
- Brains represent experiences received from our senses.

Hypnosis has many myths, not being helped by its many colourful characters throughout history but to clarify what hypnosis is. The following statement is very apt:

'Hypnosis is a completely natural state that along with the input of a properly trained and confident therapist can create positive changes in a person's mental, emotional and physical state. It cannot make you do anything that you do not want to do or that you morally object to. You cannot get stuck in hypnosis and can leave the state whenever you wish.'

*We are all different and unique!*

# 'The Dying Process— The Transition From Life to Death'

I wish to start with this chapter next on the 'dying process and the transition from life to death' before we go into any more details about hypnotherapy and the many ways it can be used. This is especially true for those who have recently been diagnosed with cancer, are coming to terms with cancer, are in hospice and palliative care (palliative care is the active care of patients with advanced progressive illness), or indeed the many carers, friends, and family who, at this time of grief, sorrow, and loss, are looking for help and answers to how to deal with these new-found emotions, feelings, and anxiety.

Quite often, many people can only release on their emotions after the person they care or love for have passed away and they are left with a big hole to fill and have the emptiness and loneliness that it brings.

Hypnotherapy can help to unravel and make sense of the many psychological, emotional, and physical symptoms associated with dying and can also be used to relieve pain in surgery; it can ease suffering and aid those in terminal illness.

By dealing with all the issues at hand at the beginning and during the dying process, and not after, so much more understanding is reached and so much less suffering is encountered, not only by those in terminal illness but also by those that are all around them.

It is worth mentioning that with all the advancement in science and medical care these days, when someone is diagnosed with cancer, it doesn't just mean death. So many people are surviving now; they are more aware of what help is out there, and the diagnosis of cancer in the early stages will give more chance of prolonged life. Hypnotherapy has a very important role to play in both the welfare of the patient and those around them.

## The journey towards death and recognising the dying process

The dying process usually begins well before death actually occurs, and death is a personal journey that each individual approaches in their own unique way. Nothing is concrete, and nothing is set in stone. There are many paths one can take on this journey, but all lead to the same destination.

As one comes close to death, a process begins—a journey from the known life of this world to the unknown of what lies ahead. As that process begins, a person starts on a mental path of discovery, comprehending that death will indeed occur and believing in their own mortality. The journey ultimately leads to the physical departure from the body.

There are milestones along this journey, and because everyone experiences death in their own unique way, not everyone will stop at each milestone. Some may only touch on a few, while another may stop at each one, taking their time in each along the way. Some may take months to reach their destination, and others will take only a few days.

We will discuss very briefly (I feel to go into great length about the dying process is beyond the scope of this book, and I encourage you, the reader, to explore this more thoroughly. There are many excellent books on the subject that have been written already) what has been found through the many researches done to establish the journey one must take, but you should always keep in mind that the journey really is subject to the individual traveller.

## The journey begins: one to three months prior to death

As people begin to accept their mortality and realise that death is approaching, they may begin to withdraw from their surroundings—they are beginning the process of separating from the world and those in it. They may decline visits from friends, neighbours, and even family members. When they do accept visitors, they may be difficult to interact with and care for—they are beginning to contemplate their life and revisit old memories.

They may be even evaluating how they have lived their life and sorting through any regrets. This is called undertaking 'the five tasks of dying', which we will look into further a bit later on.

The dying person may experience reduced appetite and weight loss as the body begins to slow down. The body doesn't need the energy from the food that it once did. The dying person may be sleeping more now and not responding and engaging in activities they once enjoyed. They no longer need the nourishment from the food they once did. The body does a wonderful thing during this time as altered body chemistry produces a mild sense of euphoria. They are neither hungry nor thirsty and are not suffering in any way by not eating. It is an expected part of the journey that they have begun.

**One to two weeks prior to death**

## Mental Changes

This is the time during the journey that one begins to sleep most of the time. Disorientation is common, and altered senses of perception can be expected. One may experience delusions, such as rearing hidden enemies or feeling invincible.

The dying person may also experience hallucinations, sometimes seeing or speaking to people that aren't there. Other times, these are people that have already died. Some may see this as the 'veil' being lifted between this life and the next. The person may pick at their sheets and clothing in a state of agitation. Movements and actions may seem aimless and make no sense to others. They are moving further away from life on this earth.

## Physical Changes

The body is having a more difficult time maintaining itself. There are signs that the body may show during this time. They are as follows:

- The body temperature lowers by a degree or more.
- The blood pressure lowers.

- The pulse becomes irregular and may slow down or speed up.
- There is increased perspiration.
- Skin colour changes as circulation becomes diminished. This is often more noticeable in the lips and the nails as they become pale and bluish.
- Breathing changes occur, often becoming more rapid and laboured. Congestion may also occur, causing a rattling sound, 'death rattle', and cough.
- Speaking decreases and eventually stops altogether.

## The journey's end: a couple of days to hours prior to death

The person is moving closer towards death. There may be a surge of energy as he or she gets nearer. He or she may want to get out of bed and talk to loved ones or ask for food after days of no appetite. The surge of energy may be quite a bit less noticeable but is usually used as a dying person's final physical expression before moving on.

The surge of energy is usually short, and the previous signs become more pronounced as death approaches. Breathing becomes more irregular and often slower. Congestion in the airway can increase and again can cause loud, rattled breathing.

Hands and feet may become blotchy and purplish (mottled). This mottling may slowly work its way up the arms and legs. Lips and nail beds become bluish or purple. The person becomes unresponsive and may have their eyes open or semi-open but not able to see their surroundings. It is widely believed that the 'hearing' is the last sense to go, so it is highly recommended that any loved ones and carers sit with and talk to the dying during this time.

Eventually, breathing will cease altogether and the heart stops. Death has then occurred.

## A note about grief and loss

We are all affected by loss and grief throughout our lives, and some of us will deal with it better than others, and during the diagnosis of cancer or terminal illness, how do you know how you are going to react until you are told of the impending diagnosis? You can only really imagine, but you won't truly know until the time comes. In helping others with hypnotherapy, it is essential that you have some understanding of grief and loss, not only for the patient but also for friends, family and so on.

It is the understanding that human beings have to go through an effective grief process in order to prevent dysfunctional, maladaptive, and unhelpful experiences in the future.

The moment we are born, we suffer loss, and that is the loss of the security and safety that our mother's womb brings, along with the separation we experience biologically from our mothers. As we grow and develop, we experience many losses of various and different types, and, eventually, we will form our concept of the permanence of death.

*During this time, we may well start to form our spiritual beliefs that may then help us to deal with losses in our lives.*

There is a grief curve that highlights what we should normally go through in grief and loss, which has been developed from studies on monkeys, children, adults, and the terminally ill.

The five stages in the grief curve are as follows:

- Shock
- Separation and pain
- Despair
- Acceptance
- Resolution and reorganisation

The time it takes us to work through this curve varies depending on the following:

- The type of loss
- The emotional attachment to the thing that we have lost
- The support we have
- The past experience of loss
- Our state of mental health
- Any other issues that happen as a result of that loss

Generally speaking, a normal period of time for an expected loss is in the region of two years, but as noticed from all the above criteria, this can vary greatly from situation to situation and from person to person. This can create many difficulties in a family which is suffering from loss, as different people will go through their grief pattern at different times and speeds, which causes conflict and misunderstanding and communication.

Below is looking at the stages in turn and a bit more detail:

- Shock—this happens shortly after the loss and is also joined by denial. The more difficult the loss is to cope and deal with the longer this stage might well last.
- Separation and pain—this stage happens when the person starts to feel the loss, and it is accompanied by a range of conflicting emotions, which cause confusion and distress.
- Despair—this is where the person is at his or her lowest and may well be accompanied by depression.
- Acceptance—it is where the person starts to accept his or her loss and is getting used to life without the person.
- Resolution and reorganisation—it is where the person has adjusted his or her life; the person or thing that he or she lost does not take up so much of his or her time or space in his or her life.

It is very possible that someone will get stuck in any one of these stages, and this is known as 'abnormal grief'. The result of this will be destructive and maladaptive behaviours, which is usually towards themselves, although other people will bear witness and experience the effect of them.

Hypnosis can be used to assist with grief and loss but should never be used without a full understanding of the process. It is of the upmost importance that the stages of grief must be worked through and not sidestepped, as ignoring them will result in psychological and even, in some cases, physical damage.

*Hypnosis can be used as a tool for coming to terms with the emotions that the person is feeling, and by accessing those emotions, hypnosis can relieve any such emotions locked in the past or present moment, reducing anxiety along the way.*

# The top five regrets of the dying

A nurse has recorded the most common regrets of the dying, and one of the greatest regrets of the dying is how little time they spent with their families, especially with their young children, compared to how much time they worked. It is really a life balance that many of us find difficult even now.

There was no mention of more sex or bungee jumps! A palliative nurse who has counselled the dying in their last days has revealed that after asking the question 'What would your biggest regret be if this was your last day of your life?' the top five regrets, and that among the top answers, from men in particular, was 'I wish I hadn't worked so hard'.

Bronnie Ware is an Australian nurse who spent several years working in palliative care, caring for patients in the last twelve weeks of their lives. She recorded their dying epiphanies in a blog called 'inspiration and chai', which gathered so much attention that she put her observations into a book, *The Top Five Regrets of the Dying*.

Bronnie writes of the phenomenal clarity of wisdom that people gain at the end of their lives and how we might learn from their wisdom. 'When questioned about any regrets they had or anything they would do differently,' she says, 'common themes surfaced again and again.'

Here are the top five regrets of the dying, as witnessed by Bronnie, and I do highly recommend that you do read her second book, *The Top Five Regrets of the Dying*.

## 1. I wish I'd had the courage to live a life true to myself, not the life others expected of me.

'This was the most common regret of all. When people realise that their life is almost over and looking back clearly on it, it is easy to see how many dreams have gone unfulfilled. Most people had not honoured even a half of their dreams and had to die knowing that it was due to choices they had made, or not made. Health brings a freedom very few realise, until they no longer have it.'

## 2. I wish I hadn't worked so hard.

'This came from every male patient that I nursed. They missed their children's youth and their partner's companionship. Women also spoke of this regret, but as most were from an older generation, many of the female patients had not been breadwinners. All of the men I nursed deeply regretted spending so much of their lives on the treadmill of a work existence.'

### 3. I'd wish I'd had the courage to express any feelings.

'Many people suppressed their feelings in order to keep peace with others. As a result, they settled for a mediocre existence and never became who they were truly capable of becoming. Many developed illnesses relating to the bitterness and resentment they carried as a result.'

### 4. I wish I had stayed in touch with my friends.

'Often they would not truly realise the full benefits of old friends until their dying weeks and it was not always possible to track them down. Many had become so caught up in their lives that they had let golden handshakes slip by over the years. There were many deep regrets about not giving friendships the time and effort that they deserved. Everyone misses their friends when they are dying.'

### 5. I wish I had let myself be happier.

'This is a surprisingly common one. Many did not realise until the end that happiness is a choice. They had stayed stuck in old patterns and habits. The so-called comfort of familiarity overflowed into their emotions, as well as their physical lives. Fear of change had them pretending to others, and to their selves, that they were content, when, deep within, they longed to laugh properly and have silliness in their life again.'

*What's your greatest regret so far, and what will you set out to achieve before you die?*

When you are on your deathbed, what others think of you is a very long way from your mind. How wonderful would it be to be able to let go and smile again, long before you are dying!

*Life is a choice it is your life so:*

*Choose consciously*

*Choose wisely*

*Choose honestly*

*Choose happiness*

*There is a Buddhist Inspiration*

When we are young and again when we are old, we depend heavily on the affection of others. Between these stages we usually feel that we can do everything without help from others, and that their attention is simply not important. But at this stage I think it is very important to keep deep human affection.

(*His Holiness the Dalai Lama*)

*You are never too young . . . , you are never too old . . . to make a difference*

*Life is not a race but a journey to be savoured each step of the way*

*Yesterday has gone*

*Tomorrow is a mystery*

*But today . . . today is a gift*

*After reading this, it is very hard to see how hypnotherapy can't help play a role in the helping and understanding of those with cancer (those terminal ill or not, or in both hospice and palliative care).*

## Hospice Care

Hospice care is end-of-life care provided by health professionals and volunteers. They give medical, psychological, and spiritual support. The goal of the care provided is to help people who are dying have peace, comfort, and dignity.

The caregivers try to control pain and other symptoms, so a person can remain as alert and comfortable as possible. Hospice programmes also provide services to support a patient's family.

Usually, a hospice patient is expected to live six months or less, and hospice care can take place:

At home

At a hospice centre

In a hospital

In a skilled nursing facility

## Cancer Care

Cancer affects different people in different ways. You may feel all sorts of emotions, anger, shock, fear, and uncertainty which are all common. At times, your cancer treatments may make you feel unwell, and you may have unwanted side effects to cope with, on top of everything else.

On some days, you may feel positive about your future—at other times, less so—but remember, you are an individual and there is neither a right nor a wrong way to feel.

At some time or another, you may have to cope with a physical problem caused by your cancer or by the treatment you are having.

There may be, for example, your treatment bringing up unwanted side effects that leave you feeling unwell, tired, or fed up. That is as follows:

- Constipation
- Diarrhoea
- Fatigue
- Mouth or eating problems
- Nausea
- Pain

## Palliative Care

Palliative care is an area of healthcare that focuses on relieving and preventing the suffering of patients. Unlike 'hospice care', palliative care medicine is appropriate for patients in all disease stages, including those undergoing treatment for curable illness and those living with chronic diseases, as well as patients who are nearing the end of life.

A multidisciplinary approach allows the palliative care team to address physical, emotional, spiritual, and social concerns that arise with advanced illness. Medications and treatments are said to have a palliative effect if they relieve symptoms without having a curative effect on the underlying disease or cause.

In effect, palliative care is specialised medical care for people with serious illness. It is focused on providing patients with relief from the symptoms, pain, and stress of an illness—whatever the progress. The goal is to improve the quality of life for both the patient and the family.

Palliative care is appropriate at any age and at any stage in a serious illness and can be provided along with curative treatment.

A World Health Organization statement describes palliative care as 'an approach that improves the quality of life of patients and their families facing the problems associated with the problems associated with life-threatening illness, through the prevention and relief of suffering by the means if early identification and the impeccable assessment and treatment of pain and other problems, physical, psychological and spiritual'.

More generally, however, the term palliative care may refer to any care that alleviates symptoms, whether or not there is hope of a cure by other means; thus palliative care treatments may be used to alleviate the side effects of curative treatments, such as the relieving of nausea associated with chemotherapy.

The term *palliative care* is increasingly used with regard to diseases other than cancer, such as chronic, progressive pulmonary disorders, renal disease, chronic heart failure, HIV or AIDS, and progressive neurological conditions.

In addition, the rapidly growing field of paediatric palliative care has clearly shown the need for services geared specifically for children with serious illness.

Palliative care

- Provides relief from pain, shortness of breath, nausea and other distressing symptoms
- Affirms life and regards dying as a normal process
- Intends neither to hasten nor to postpone death
- Integrates the psychological and spiritual aspects of patient care
- Offers a support system to help patients live as actively as possible

- Offers a support system to help the family cope
- Uses a team approach to address the needs of patients and their families
- Will enhance quality of life
- Is applicable early in the course of illness, in conjunction with other therapies that are intended to prolong life

While palliative care may seem to offer a broad range of services, the goals of palliative care treatment are concrete: relief from suffering, treatment of pain and other distressing symptoms, psychological and spiritual care, a support system to help the individual live as actively as possible, and a rapport system to sustain and rehabilitate the individual's family.

# How can hypnotherapy help with cancer?

The use of hypnotherapy has gained wide acceptance in helping patients cope with the diagnosis and treatment of cancer. When someone is diagnosed with cancer, the fear of the unknown begins to take over, both for the family and the patient. This alone in itself can contribute to an enormous level of anxiety and worry on top of the normal stresses of day-to-day life.

Many times, when someone faces the prospect of medical treatment, they will feel a sense of helplessness and a loss of control over his or her own life. Hypnosis is a powerful tool for creating new, more effective coping mechanisms to manage these stresses with a sense of control while in the healing process.

The primary goal of hypnosis as a complement to medical cancer therapies is to return to the patient a feeling of control and a greater understanding of the body-mind connection. This creates the best holistic combination medicine can offer, coupled with the power of the subconscious mind. When someone faces a serious illness from an understanding that they are in control and are empowered by their medical treatment, the prospect of success, as well as their sense of overall well-being, is greatly improved.

Regaining all important sense of control and reducing the associated stress and anxiety of coping with cancer allows the perspective of hopelessness to become one of hopefulness.

Hypnotherapy can be used to help those suffering from cancer in many ways such as follows:

- Overcoming fears and phobias
- Fear of surgery
- Fear of hospitals
- Fear of radiotherapy
- Fear of chemotherapy

Reducing or eliminating side effects such as follows:

- Pain
- Nausea
- Sleeplessness
- Fatigue
- Bowel habit disturbance
- Learning to visualise boosting the immune system and fighting the disease
- Controlling levels of pain and discomfort

Emotional and psychological such as follows:

- Recognising and acknowledging feelings around diagnosis
- Recognising feelings of control
- Working through feelings about loss
- Diagnosis support
- Learning to relax body and be kind to their own body

It is very important to stress that a cancer patient can become proactive with his or her disease by using hypnosis and guided imagery to get in touch with his or her immune system. Through hypnosis, a patient can visualise his or her body fighting the cancer, becoming healthier and removing the invader. During hypnosis, he or she is able to 'see' the chemotherapy drugs doing their job and help his or her body eliminate the toxins from his or her system.

There are many examples of the possibilities used from hypnosis; however, the most effective suggestions are tailored specifically to the individual's needs (something we will go in to more detail later on in this book), personal preferences, and the way he or she individually processes language. Once a patient has experienced deep trance states of guided hypnosis a number of times, techniques of self-hypnosis are easily taught. Hypnosis then becomes a tool that can be used at any time to facilitate recovery.

So, for example, if someone believed he or she could see, feel, and taste the cool refreshment of a mint leaf whenever he or she were beginning to experience the unpleasant feeling of nausea, that new sensation would replace the unwanted sensation. Or, if one were to imagine their favourite place, a beautiful high mountain lake, surrounded by peaceful high mountains, sitting comfortably enjoying the experience, he or she would not notice the discomfort of the needle in his or her physical body because a pleasant detachment has taken place. A patient may be aware of some pressure, but he or she will not experience the pain, anxiety, and tension associated with the procedure.

This happens because we experience our world through our five senses. Information we receive stimulates certain areas of the brain; it is then processed and is then sent to the areas that control higher functions. When someone is hypnotised and given suggestions of imagery while their brain is being scanned, areas of the brain are stimulated as if they were actually experiencing the events of the guided imagery. In other words, the mind does not seem to know the difference what is perceived by our senses and what our imagination can experience in the deeply relaxed states of hypnotherapy. Our physiology will respond in the same way as if we were truly experiencing the changes in the environment.

Because hypnotherapy seeks to support and complement (and not replace) mainstream medical treatments, it is a powerful tool, and when illness occurs in the physical body, it is important to recognise that it has been present in the 'mental plane' as a negative thought and emotion pattern for a long period of time.

Another way to look at this repetitive pattern, which has led to a bodily breakdown, is to see it requiring a combination of intervention through the following:

- Mainstream medicine, which is to address the 'hardware'—the physical body
- Complementary approaches like hypnotherapy to address the 'software'—mental and emotional aspects

It is important to note that even if the same 'software' continues to run on a new 'hardware' (healed physical body), recurrence of the illness is likely.

At the emotional or mental level, hypnotherapy would focus on the following:

- Tracing the origin of the guilt and releasing it through 'inner child work'
- Releasing the residual emotional change of traumatic memories
- Reigniting the mind's capacity to guide the individual's own healing through guided imagery
- Improving the quality of life (even if 'quality of life' cannot be enhanced) by coaching the individual to reach a place of acceptance in the here and now

## How can hypnotherapy help with hospice and palliative care?

Knowing that you have a terminal illness can take a heavy toll on both the patient and family, friends, loved ones, and partners. It is never going to be an easy time for anybody, but with the help of those working in a hospice or in a palliative care setting, and with the support network surrounding it, there is much valuable help available.

There are many emotions and feelings that can come up at such times, and they all need to be dealt with in the appropriate way and manner. Left untreated, it can cause immense suffering for everyone concerned, not only in the process of dying but in aftercare afterwards.

At an onset of a diagnosis of terminal illness, it can take a heavy toll and many emotions and feelings can come to the surface, such as anger, depression, anxiety, and regret. All these feelings can impair the ability to cope with diagnoses as effectively as possible.

It is imperative to know that you can reconcile your emotions and still enjoy life and the time you have while going through treatment.

By using hypnotherapy in hospice and palliative care, it has proved to be very successful in helping people to adapt and manage both themselves and their families as effectively as possible.

By addressing their personal issues and exploring relationship resolution, people in palliative care can enjoy each day so much more.

Many patients in palliative care dislike the perception of not being in control, and they have received huge amounts of attention, treatment, and resources but feel outside the loop. With the help of hypnotherapy, it can help the patient take more responsibility for their condition (if they wish to), and regular positive action can be taken in between the many and, sometimes, endless medical appointments.

Hypnosis and, more importantly, self-hypnosis, has a vital role to play. The two main ones being relaxation and an establishment of a stronger mind or body link.

## Relaxation

Many patients have had difficulty in relaxing deeply, sometimes for all their lives. Hypnosis provides a welcome relief, and the benefits can be practiced at home in the form of self-hypnosis. Just ten or twenty minutes every day can bring great benefits, with feelings of calm and higher self-esteem.

## Boosting the immune system

Processes to boost the immune system can also be practiced at home in the state of deep relaxation. A growing area of study carries the rather cumbersome title of Psychoneuroimmunology (PNI). Research in PNI has shown that a person in a good mood can produce more white blood corpuscles than that same person in a bad mood, thus increasing their potential to fight disease.

Mental work is done by the patient to increase awareness of the presence of the circulatory and immune systems. Patients develop very personal ways to imagine the process, and time spent strengthening the neural pathways between the mind and body is never wasted.

## Symptom relief

Hypnosis can also help in the relief of some of the symptoms associated with palliative care, for example, sleep disturbance, anger, pain, lethargy, and guilt. Hypnosis can introduce new and positive ways to tackle old challenges.

There has much research been done in the effectiveness of hypnotherapy in the treatment with cancer patients receiving palliative care. I wish to quote the following from one of these, being from the BMJ:

'The study into hypnotherapy and supportive and palliative care suggests that hypnotherapy can contribute in anxiety in palliative care patients with the added benefit of improving sleep and severity of psychological and physical symptoms.'

Most chronic illnesses, including cancer and heart disease, are complex—having more than one cause and often more than one treatment. The medical teams work very hard to treat the disease, but often the patient gets trapped on a medical 'treadmill' without the peace and quiet they need, to consider their own needs.

Patients suffering from these serious conditions also have all the small niggles that the rest of us do—headache, stomach upset, coughs and colds, dental pain, and so on, and it is often these small things which can really bring a person down. So there is a real benefit in investigating early on in diagnosis in a plan for managing ongoing symptoms, medical interventions, and the emotional side effects of chronic illness; hypnotherapy can help with this.

I would like to give you, the reader, some examples of hypnotherapy scripts, which will give you an idea of how it can relate to cancer, hospice, and palliative care.

After these, I will then move on how to write your own scripts and how you can personalise them to suit each individual case and issue at hand.

# Relaxation

**Script . . .**

You are sitting here today . . . in this very special chair . . . and today . . . today this chair will allow you to be more comfortable . . . more comfortable than you have ever felt before . . . you feel calm and relaxed . . . relaxed and calm . . .

Now . . . now you may wish to close your eyes . . . or wait . . . or wait until they become heavier and heavier . . . heavier and heavier and wish to close all by themselves . . . you feel calm and relaxed . . . relaxed and calm . . .

And because you feel calm and relaxed . . . , you find it easy to concentrate on my voice . . . to listen to my voice . . . , and as you listen to my voice more and more . . . , all other sounds inside and outside this room slowly begin to disappear . . . calm and relaxed . . . relaxed and calm . . .

The more you listen to my voice . . . , the more relaxed you feel . . . , and as you listen to my voice, you notice you are concentrating on your breath . . . You are concentrating on your breathing . . . and as you breathe in, your belly rises . . . and as you breathe out, your belly falls . . . Breathe in belly rise . . . Breath out belly fall . . . Breath in belly rise . . . Breath out belly fall . . . Calm and relaxed . . . Relaxed and calm . . .

Relax . . . relax . . . relax . . .

Breathe in belly rise . . . Breathe out belly fall . . . Breathe in belly rise . . . Breathe out belly fall . . .

Calm and relaxed . . . Relaxed and calm . . .

Relax . . . relax . . . relax . . .

And as you continue to relax . . . more and more . . . more and more . . . , you begin to relax the muscles in your whole body . . . from the tips of your toes to the top of your head . . . You relax the muscles in your whole body . . . so now let's start with the muscles in your toes . . .

Relax your toes . . . relax your toes . . . relax your toes . . .
Relax your feet . . . relax your feet . . . relax your feet . . .
Relax your ankles . . . relax your ankles . . . relax your ankles . . .
Relax . . . relax . . . relax . . .
Relax your calves . . . relax your calves . . . relax your calves . . .
Relax your knees . . . relax your knees . . . relax your knees . . .
Relax your legs . . . relax your legs . . . relax your legs . . .
Relax . . . relax . . . relax . . .
Relax your thighs . . . relax your thighs . . . relax your thighs . . .
Relax your hips . . . relax your hips . . . relax your hips . . .
Relax your stomach . . . relax your stomach . . . relax your stomach . . .
Relax . . . relax . . . relax . . .
Relax your chest . . . relax your chest . . . relax your chest . . .
Relax your back . . . relax your back . . . relax your back . . .
Relax . . . relax . . . relax . . .
Relax your arms . . . relax your arms . . . relax your arms . . .
Relax your fingers . . . relax your fingers . . . relax your fingers . . .
Relax your shoulders . . . relax your shoulders . . . relax your shoulders . . .
Relax . . . relax . . . relax . . .
Relax your neck . . . relax your neck . . . relax your neck . . .
Relax your head . . . relax your head . . . relax your head . . .
Relax your face . . . relax your face . . . relax your face . . .
Relax your eyes . . . relax your eyes . . . relax your eyes . . .
Deeply relaxed . . . deeply . . . deeply relaxed . . .

And as you relax more and more . . . more and more . . . , you allow your mind to drift . . . You allow your mind to slowly . . . gently . . . calmly . . . drift . . . drift . . . drift . . . drift . . .

And now . . . and now as you allow your mind to drift . . . , I would like you to imagine that you are standing at a top of a set of stairs . . . , and these stairs lead you down to a wonderful place . . . a wonderful special place . . . a landscape of vast beauty . . . a place of total peace and serenity . . . a place where you feel so safe . . . a place where you feel calm and safe . . . safe and calm . . . nobody needs anything from you . . . and nobody wants anything from you . . . This is your special place . . . your very own special place . . .

And this place can be somewhere that you have been before . . . It can be somewhere that you would like to go . . . or it can be somewhere . . . somewhere that your mind does really imagine . . . Choose this place . . . Choose this place . . . This really is your very own special place . . .

And now . . . now as you see yourself standing at the top of the set of stairs . . . , you notice there is a firm handrail . . . , you feel safe and protected . . . protected and safe . . . , you hold on to that handrail and you see ten steps leading down . . . , leading down to your very own special place . . .

And when you are ready . . . when you are ready . . . , you begin to walk down those steps . . . slowly . . . one step at a time . . . ready now . . .

Ten . . . going down . . . deeper and deeper . . . deeper and deeper . . .
Nine . . . going down . . . deeper and deeper . . . deeper and deeper . . .
Eight . . . going down . . . deeper still . . . deeper . . . deeper still . . .
Seven . . . down you go . . . deeper . . . deeper . . . deeper . . .
Six . . . going down . . . saying to yourself . . . I am calm . . . I feel calm . . . I am calm . . . I feel calm . . .
Five . . . going down . . . deeper and deeper . . . deeper and deeper . . .
Four . . . down you go . . . deeper . . . deeper still . . .
Three . . . two . . . one . . . down you go . . . deeper . . . deeper . . . deeper . . .
Deeper relaxed . . . deeper . . . deeper . . . relaxed . . .

Now . . . now you find yourself at the bottom of the set of stairs . . . and at the bottom of the set of stairs . . . , you notice a large oak door . . . , and you begin to walk towards that door . . . In your hand, you have a key . . . a key to unlock that door . . . You walk towards that door . . . and you put the key into the lock . . . You turn the key . . . , and you gently push the door open . . . The door opens slowly . . . and you then push that door a little harder . . . and you begin to walk through that door . . .

And as you go through that large oak door, you marvel at the beauty of your very own special place . . . You feel calm and relaxed here . . . relaxed and calm . . . , and as you are now in your very own special place . . . , I will leave you here for a short while . . . a short while to explore . . . to enjoy the feelings . . . that your very own special place brings you . . . , and when you next hear my voice . . . , I will gently . . . slowly . . . bring you back . . . I will count down from ten to one . . . , and when I reach one . . . , you will be able to open your eyes . . . and all other sounds . . . inside . . . and outside this room . . . will become aware to you . . .

Pause . . . one to two minutes . . .

It is now time to come back to the room . . . And you will bring back with you all the feelings of peace and calm . . . that your very own special place brings you . . . and remember . . . remember, you can come back to this place any time you wish . . . Ready now . . .

Ten . . . nine . . . waking up now . . . waking up now . . .
Eight . . . seven . . . waking up . . . waking up now . . .
Six . . . five . . . waking up . . . you feel the ground beneath your feet . . .
Four . . . three . . . wide awake now . . . wide awake now . . .
Two . . . one . . . wide awake . . . wide awake now . . .
Welcome back . . .

# Dying Regrets

**Script...**

And now . . . now as you begin to drift deeper and deeper . . . deeper and deeper . . . , you feel calm and relaxed . . . relaxed and calm . . . You are here in your very own special place . . .

I would now like you . . . to become aware of the time of the day . . . the time of the year . . . and feel . . . feel the position of your body resting here in space . . . , and there is no place for you to go right now . . . There is no problem that you need to solve . . . There is nothing to do but relax . . . relax and let go . . . let go and relax . . .

You are now deeply relaxed . . . deeply relaxed . . . , and the suggestions that you will hear . . . will hear from the sound of my voice . . . will have an immediate and permanent effect on your subconscious mind . . . You will hear every word that I speak . . . and even though you may find your mind wandering away at times . . . , nothing else matters . . . except for this wonderful feeling of relaxation that you are feeling . . .

And now . . . now I want you to imagine a large oak door in front of you . . . and you walk towards that door . . . In your hand is a key . . . , and you put the key into the lock of that door . . . You gently push the door . . . and it begins to slowly open . . . and you now push that door a bit harder and the door opens wider . . . even further . . . and you now walk through that door . . . In front of you is a chair . . . Next to the chair is a desk . . .

You sit down on that chair . . . You feel calm and relaxed . . . relaxed and calm . . .

And resting on that desk is a book . . . a book with the title *Dying Regrets . . . the Top Five Regrets of the Dying* . . . You are intrigued by the title of that book . . . and you open that book . . . and you begin reading . . . and you begin to read the words . . .

The words . . . 'What would your biggest regret be if this was your last day of your life?' . . .

Pause fifteen seconds . . .

You now begin to carry on reading that book further . . . even further . . . , and you read the words . . . You read the words . . .

An Australian nurse spent several years working in palliative care . . . caring for patients in the last twelve weeks of their lives . . . and she recorded their dying words in a book . . . a book titled, *Dying Regrets . . . the Top Five Regrets of the Dying* . . . and the nurse wrote the phenomenal clarity of wisdom . . . that people gain at the end of their lives . . . and how we might learn from their wisdom . . . , and when questioned about any regrets they had or anything they would do differently . . . , they replied with the following . . .

The following top five regrets of the dying . . .

Pause ten seconds . . .

One . . .

I wish I had the courage to live a life true to myself . . . and not the life others expected of me . . .

I wish I had the courage to live a life true to myself . . . and not the life others expected of me . . .

I wish I had the courage to live a life true to myself . . . and not the life others expected of me . . .

Pause ten seconds . . .

This is the most common regret of all . . . when people realise their life is almost over . . . and look back clearly on it . . . , it is easy to see how many dreams have gone unfulfilled . . . Many people had not even honoured even a half of their dreams . . . and had to die . . . knowing that it was due to choices they had made, or not made . . . Health brings a freedom very few realise . . . until they no longer have it . . .

Pause ten seconds . . .

Two . . .

I wish I hadn't worked so hard . . .
I wish I hadn't worked so hard . . .
I wish I hadn't worked so hard . . .

Pause ten seconds . . .

This came from every male patient that I nursed . . . They missed their children's youth . . . and their partner's companionship . . . Women also spoke of this regret . . . , but as many were from an older generation . . . , many of them had not been breadwinners . . . But they all deeply regretted spending so much of their lives on the treadmill of a work existence . . .

Pause ten seconds . . .

Three . . .

I wish I had the courage to express my feelings . . .
I wish I had the courage to express my feelings . . .
I wish I had the courage to express my feelings . . .

Pause ten seconds . . .

Many people suppressed their feelings in order to keep peace with others . . . , and as a result, they settled for a mediocre existence and never became who they were truly capable of becoming . . . many developed illnesses relating to the bitterness and resentment they carried as a result . . .

Pause ten seconds . . .

Four . . .

I wish I had stayed in touch with my friends . . .
I wish I had stayed in touch with my friends . . .

I wish I had stayed in touch with my friends . . .

Pause ten seconds . . .

Often they would not truly realise the full benefits of old friends until their dying weeks . . . and it was not always possible to track them down . . . Many had been so caught up in their lives . . . and they had deep regrets about not giving friendship the time and effort that they deserved . . . Everyone misses their friends when they are dying . . .

Pause ten seconds . . .

Five . . .

I wish I had let myself be happier . . .
I wish I had let myself be happier . . .
I wish I had let myself be happier . . .

Pause ten seconds . . .

This is a surprisingly common one . . . Many did not realise until the end . . . that happiness is a choice . . . They had stayed stuck in old patterns and habits . . . and had stayed in their comfort zone . . . not expanding their emotional and physical lives . . . and fear of change had them pretending to others, to their selves, that they were content . . . when deep within, they longed to laugh properly and have silliness in their life again . . .

Pause ten seconds . . .

Now . . . now you know what the biggest regrets are of those that were dying . . . , how does that make you feel . . . ?

Pause ten seconds . . .

Some of these regrets . . . may not be those that you are thinking right now . . . , but when you are on your deathbed . . . , what will *your* regrets be . . . ?

Pause twenty seconds . . .

And now . . . now as you close the book . . . and put it back on the table . . . , I want you to ask yourself a question . . . 'What is my greatest regret in life . . . so far? . . . And what will I set out to achieve before I die . . . ?'

I will leave you for a short while to ask yourself those questions . . . , and when you next hear my voice . . . , I will bring you back . . . slowly . . . gently back . . .

Pause ninety seconds . . .

Bring back . . .

# The Dying Process: The Transition From Life to Death

**Script . . .**

As you begin to drift deeper and deeper . . . deeper and deeper . . . , you find yourself at the bottom of the set of stairs . . . , you feel calm and relaxed . . . relaxed and calm . . . , you notice a large . . . old . . . oak door . . . just ahead of you . . . , and you walk towards that door . . . The door is locked . . . , but you are holding a key in your hand . . . You put the key into the lock . . . and the door slowly opens . . . You walk through that door . . . into your very own special place . . . a place where you feel calm and relaxed . . . relaxed and calm . . .

You find a comfortable place to sit . . . and you sit down . . . listening to the sound of my voice more and more . . . more and more . . . deeply relaxed . . . deeply relaxed . . .

And now . . . now I would like to thank you for coming here today . . . for listening to this hypnotic CD . . . I respect and honour you for being here . . . today . . . I know this is a very difficult time for you right now . . . You have learned recently that you are terminally ill . . . and you are probably going through a whole range of unwanted emotions right now . . .

It is understandable . . . that you may feel sad . . . for death seems so final . . . and I am sure you would give anything you could . . . in order to keep yourself . . .

your body alive . . . , but, of course, deep inside . . . you know that it is not possible . . .

You are here today . . . to learn of the process . . . to learn of the dying process . . . to learn of the transition from life to death . . . to learn that dying . . . dying really is a part of living . . . a part of life . . . something that we all . . . we all face at one point in our life . . .

It is said . . . It is said that there are several stages of grieving . . . sorrow . . . that your time is coming to an end . . .

Stage one . . . denial . . .
Stage two . . . anger . . .
Stage three . . . bargaining . . .
Stage four . . . depression . . .
Stage five . . . acceptance . . .

And because you . . . and any of your loved ones are already going through these grieving processes . . . , I want you to realise . . . to realise that you *will* reach that last stage of acceptance . . . to reach that last stage before your death . . . to have that acceptance that everything will be OK . . . that everything is OK . . .

So now . . . now I would like you to imagine that your arms are outstretched . . . and your pals are facing up . . . and as you do so . . . , I want you to think the following words in your mind . . . 'I accept that this is going to happen . . . and I accept that this will probably happen soon . . .'

And . . . and as you do so, I would like you to remember the words . . . remember the words . . . 'I want to hold you till I die . . . till we both break down and cry . . . and I want to hold you till the fears in me subside . . .'

Now . . . now I want you to realise that death is a personal journey . . . a death . . . that each one of us . . . approaches in his or her own individual and unique way . . . and remember that nothing is concrete . . . nothing is set in stone . . . and that there are many paths one can take on this journey of ours . . . but . . . but all paths . . . all roads . . . all journeys . . . lead to the same destination . . .

And as one comes close to death . . . , a process begins . . . a journey from the known life of this world . . . to the unknown that lies ahead . . . and as that process begins . . . , a person starts on a mental part of discovery . . . which . . .

which comprehends that death will occur . . . , and the journey . . . ultimately leads to the physical departure of the body . . .

There are many milestones along this journey . . . , and because everyone experiences death in their own unique way . . . , not everyone will stop at each milestone . . . Some may only touch on a few . . . while another may stop at each one . . . taking their time in each along the way . . . , and some . . . some may take many months to reach their destination . . . while others . . . others will take only a few days . . .

And remember . . . remember that everyone is different and unique . . . We are all unique and different . . .

Now . . . now the journey begins one to three months prior to death . . . , and as you begin to accept that death is approaching . . . , you may begin to withdraw from your surroundings . . . You are beginning the process of separating from the world . . . and those that are in it . . . , and you may . . . you may even decline visits . . . from loved ones . . . , friends . . . , neighbours . . . , family members . . .

You may find that when you do accept visitors . . . , you may find it difficult to interact . . . to talk with them . . . and then . . . you may begin to contemplate your life . . . and revisit old memories . . . You may be looking at how you lived your life . . . and maybe even going through any regrets . . .

The dying person may . . . may experience reduced appetite and weight loss . . . as the body begins to slow down . . . The body doesn't need the energy from the food it once did . . . You may find that you are sleeping more now . . . and not responding and engaging in activities that you once enjoyed . . . You no longer need the nourishment from food . . . that you once did . . .

And you know . . . you know that the body does a wonderful thing during this time . . . as the altered body chemistry produces a mild sense of euphoria . . . You are neither hungry nor thirsty . . . , and you are not suffering in any way by not eating . . . It is an expected part of the journey that you have begun . . .

And now . . . now one to two weeks before death . . . This is the time that you begin to sleep most of the time . . . You may become disorientated and may experience delusions, . . . such as facing hidden enemies or feeling invincible . . . You may even experience seeing or speaking to people who are not in the room with you . . . You may even feel agitated . . . , and your movements may seem aimless and make no sense to others . . .

At this point in time, you are moving further away from life on this earth . . . and the body may be having a difficult time maintaining itself . . . Your body may be showing signs at this time . . . such as . . . the body temperature dropping a degree or two . . . , blood pressure lowering . . . , the pulse becoming irregular . . . slowing down or speeding up . . .

You may also find there is increased perspiration . . . and the skin colour changes . . . as your circulation becomes diminished . . . You may even find the lips and the nails become pale and bluish . . .

Breathing changes may occur . . . becoming more rapid and laboured . . . Congestion in the throat may cause a cough and a rattling sound . . . while speech decreases and eventually stops altogether . . .

And now . . . now the journey comes to an end . . . and a couple of days to hours prior to death . . . , you will be moving nearer and nearer to death . . . and as you do . . . , you may find a sudden urge of energy as you get nearer . . . and nearer . . . nearer and nearer . . . You may even want to climb out of bed and talk to loved ones . . . or even ask for food after days of no appetite . . .

This sudden surge of energy is usually short . . . and the previous signs become more pronounced as death approaches . . . Breathing becomes more irregular . . . and often slower . . . hands and feet may become blotchy and purplish . . . and this mottling may slowly work its way up to the arms and legs . . .

Lips and nail beds bluish or become purple . . . , and you may find you become unresponsive . . . Your eyes open or semi-open but not able to see your surroundings . . .

It is widely believed that the hearing is the last sense to go . . . , and it is highly recommended that any loved ones . . . any carers . . . sit and talk with you at this time . . . and . . . and as your breathing begins to slow down . . . , I want you to remember these words . . . to remember the words . . . 'I want to hold you till I die . . . to reach out and cry . . . 'and as you do so, you hear the words playing in the background . . . 'I want to hold you till I die . . . till we both break down and cry . . . and I want to hold you till the fears in me subside . . .'

Pause twenty seconds . . .

And now . . . now you have no regrets . . . You are at peace . . . You are at one with yourself . . . You know now the dying process . . . , and however it is for you . . . , it is fine . . . It is perfectly fine . . .

It is now time to come back to the room . . .

Bring gently back . . .

# Loss of a Loved One

**Script . . .**

And now . . . now as you go deeper and deeper . . . deeper and deeper . . . , you find yourself in your special place . . . your very own special place . . . you feel calm and safe . . . safe and calm . . .

You feel at peace here in your very own special place . . . and you marvel at all the beauty that is all around you . . . the vivid colours . . . the sounds of the beautiful creatures in the sky . . . on the ground . . . in the sea . . . This is a magical place . . . your very own special magical place . . .

And because you feel protected and safe . . . safe and protected . . . , we are here today . . . this very moment in time . . . to talk about things . . . to talk about things that maybe are not so easy to talk about . . . the things that you have been holding on to for a very long time . . .

And because . . . because losing someone we love . . . losing someone we love . . . really is the most difficult thing that we have to live through . . . , it doesn't matter if you have only known this person for a short while . . . or known them for a very long time . . . The feelings are all the same . . . The feelings of sorrow . . . grief . . . and loss are all the same . . .

I know . . . I know that at this present moment . . . , this present moment in time . . . in your life . . . you may be experiencing many unhappy feelings . . . that are hard . . . that are hard to bear . . . I want you to know . . . to know that we all go through the grieving process in our own unique way . . . , and at the moment . . . this moment in time . . . , you may feel that you are in a dark tunnel . . . which appears to have no end . . .

Do you know . . . do you know that they say there are five stages of grief . . . that there are five stages of grief that we all go through . . . at a time of loss . . . ?

And they are . . . they are . . .

One . . .

Slight pause . . .
Denial . . . that this cannot be happening to me . . . this cannot be happening to me . . . this cannot be happening to me . . .
Slight pause . . .

Two . . .

Slight pause . . .
Anger . . . Why is this happening to me . . . ? Who is to blame . . . ? Why is this happening to me . . . ? Who is to blame . . . ? Why is this happening to me . . . ? Who is to blame . . . ?

Slight pause . . .

Three . . .
Slight pause . . .
Bargaining . . . Make this not happen and in return I will . . . make this not happen and in return I will . . . make this not happen and in return I will . . .
Slight pause . . .

Four . . .
Slight pause . . .
Depression . . . I am sad to do anything . . . I am sad to do anything . . . I am sad to do anything . . .
Slight pause . . .

Five . . .
Slight pause . . .
Acceptance . . . I am at peace with myself . . . I am at peace with myself . . . I am at peace with myself . . .
Slight pause . . .

Now . . . you need to remember . . . you need to remember that not everyone who is grieving . . . goes through all these stages . . . and that's OK . . . for you do not have to go through each stage in order to heal . . .

You may find that any emotions that you are feeling may even change from day to day . . . They can change from denial to guilt . . . from anger to acceptance . . . , and do you know . . . do you know that some people may not feel any emotion at all . . . ? It is as though a part of them has died as well . . .

You may feel at times that you can't go on without the person that you lost . . . but . . . but these feelings are perfectly normal . . .

We can ask ourselves . . . why did this happen? . . . What is the point of living? . . . What could I have done to prevent this happening? . . . We may even feel angry that they left us . . . and again, this is part of the grieving process . . .

Only you know what you are feeling right now . . . and I want you to know that whatever you are feeling . . . whatever you are feeling right now is perfectly OK . . . perfectly OK . . .

I know . . . and you know . . . that you loved this person . . . and . . . and you still do . . . and I am sure that you always will . . . I want you to remember . . . to remember that no one can ever take that away from you . . . and if you ever feel like crying . . . or screaming . . . or shouting . . . , then that is what you must do . . . It is perfectly fine to do so . . . It is perfectly fine to do so . . .

So now . . . now please do not bottle those feelings up . . . for they are an expression . . . an expression of your feeling of loss . . . and the love that you have for your dearly departed one . . .

Now . . . now sometimes when someone dies . . . , we can be upset for ourselves . . . and it is our loss that we feel . . . , but I want you to remember . . . to remember that your parent . . . your friend . . . your partner . . . your husband . . . your wife . . . or whoever that person is . . . is at peace . . . is really so much at peace . . .

They may have been suffering . . . and you may have been watching them suffering . . . , but that suffering is over now . . . and they will not have to go through that suffering any more . . .

Now . . . now whatever your belief system is . . . , there is one thing for certain . . . that there is a beginning and an end to our life on this earth . . . The cycles of nature continue forever . . . as the buds in spring form on a shrub and unfold into a beautiful flower . . . which opens up to the summer sun . . . and turns brown with the autumn breeze . . . before leaving its life and fluttering to the ground . . . and that leaf or flower will go back to where it came from . . . the earth . . . mother earth . . .

Now . . . now the memories that you hold in your heart are precious . . . , and although the person you love is not here in a physical sense . . . , your memories in your heart will be with you forever . . . , and remember . . . remember, your memories are like beautiful jewels . . . You can take them out and look at them . . . and feel the presence of your departed loved one in you . . .

You can feel that calm acceptance . . . beginning . . . beginning to replace those conflicting emotions . . . , and even as you are listening to the sound of my voice . . . , you are already beginning to feel calmer . . . and that life is becoming brighter as you see the light at the end of the tunnel . . . You may . . . you may still have a little way to go . . . , but the light is there and gets brighter and brighter day by day . . .

I want you now . . . I want you now to feel the burden that you have been carrying . . . now lifting away from you . . . and you feel your heart becoming lighter and lighter . . . and as that calm acceptance begins to spread throughout your body . . . , your whole self also becomes lighter and lighter . . . lighter and lighter . . .

And . . . and now I want you to remember that each and every one of us is different . . . unique . . . and special . . . for we all deal and cope . . . with life in our own special way . . . There is no right way . . . There is no wrong way . . . All there is . . . all there is . . . is your way . . . and whichever way you choose to cope with life . . . and its ups and downs . . . is perfectly fine . . . It is perfectly fine . . .

And now . . . now every day becomes a little easier for you to bear . . . , and each and every day, you are moving further and further towards the light . . . further and further . . . to becoming whole again . . . just like your dearly departed one would have wanted you to do . . .

Now . . . now remember that you carry all those treasures within your heart . . . and even though you may never forget . . . , you will be able to see each and every day with a new purpose . . . a new way of being . . . to becoming whole again . . . becoming whole again . . .

Pause ten seconds . . .

Bring safely back . . .

One of the aspects of cancer that most people are afraid of is the treatment and all its side effects. It is very important to use hypnosis in conjunction and alongside the treatment plan and not as a substitute for medical help.

The following scripts are intended for relaxation purposes only and are not a medical or therapeutic device and is not intended to diagnose, treat, cure, or prevent any medical condition or disease.

# Living With Cancer: Relaxation for Chemotherapy

**Script...**

Now . . . now you are in your special place . . . safe and secure . . . secure and safe . . . I would like you to recall and remember . . . remember the discussions that you have had with doctors . . . the surgeons . . . about the treatment that is going to take place for you . . .

They have explained to you about chemotherapy . . . and all the possible side effects . . . and you understand all this . . . You understand all this . . .

So now . . . now when you go for your chemotherapy . . . , you can empty your mind . . . empty your mind of any distracting . . . thoughts . . . worries . . . concerns . . . and you can concentrate on yourself . . . the self-hypnosis that you have learned . . . to complement the treatment . . . that the doctors . . . surgeons . . . nurses are going to give to you . . . You are happy . . . to allow all those doctors . . . nurses . . . surgeons . . . do what it is they are best trained to do . . .

And now . . . right now . . . , at this present moment . . . , you are ready to tackle . . . those cancer cells that are invading your body . . . and you are ready to fight these cells . . .

You know that you are a fighter . . . a fighter to do battle . . . and you are going to fight that cancer every step of the way . . . using your very own imagination to heal the body . . . and you know . . . that you can put up with a bit of disruption in your life . . . if you know that this will help you in your battle . . . your very own battle . . .

Now . . . now I want you to know that some of these powerful medicines may try to play tricks on your body . . . , but you are ready for them if they do . . . because you know now that this is just a possible reaction that your body may have to the drugs . . . and that's OK . . . because you know that the main thing is that those drugs are there to kill off those cancer cells . . .

And one of the sensations may be the feeling of something in your stomach that shouldn't be there . . . , but you know that in reality, everything is exactly how it should be . . .

Now . . . now you are prepared . . . for if your body is fooled into thinking there is something there that shouldn't be . . . , you are prepared . . .

You can . . . and will be able to relax your whole body . . . just like you have done today . . . I would now like you to concentrate on your hands . . . Which one of those hands do you use the most? Which one of those hands is the one you rely on the most . . . ?

Now you know which hand this is . . . I would like you to imagine a warm and tingly sensation flowing through that hand . . . You could possibly imagine that you are warming your hands by a blazing log fire . . . on a cold winter's day . . . and you feel that heat spreading into your hand . . . your palm . . . your fingers . . .

And now . . . now when you can feel that warmth . . . , you can bring your hand up . . . and place it on to your stomach . . . and you can feel the sensations just easing and melting away . . . just melting and soothing and easing away . . . You can feel the relief that it brings to you . . .

Now some people . . . some people say they experience a strange taste in their mouth . . . and that's OK . . . It is just a taste . . . and should your body ever think it can taste something that shouldn't be there . . . , you are ready for it . . . You could imagine a fresh lemon . . . being cut into slices . . . and as you are cutting the lemon . . . , you can see the juice beginning to squirt out of the lemon . . .

And now . . . now I want you to imagine putting that lemon to your mouth . . . and that lemon begins to cleanse your mouth . . . to make it feel clean once more . . . and the nasty taste that was there before is replaced . . . replaced by the tangy . . . clean . . . juicy . . . lemon taste . . .

And now . . . now if you feel nauseous sometimes . . . , I would like you to ride with it . . . I want you to imagine you are on a ship . . . on a ship riding the ocean waves . . . You are on top of the waves . . . and you are the captain of the ship . . . You are in control . . . and the waves do not bother you . . . because you know the waves will pass . . . and if there is ever . . . ever anything that needs to be brought up . . . from inside your stomach . . . , it will be brought up . . . because you know that when you are sick . . . sick from the inside . . . , you know that it is your own body's way of realising what it needs to . . . It will bring up all what it needs to . . . to make you feel better . . . and you know that you do feel much better for bringing it all up . . .

Some people may experience hair loss . . . with chemotherapy . . . and once again . . . you do not mind this . . . You really do not mind this . . . because you know . . . you know that it means that those wonderful drugs . . . are working inside you . . . inside you . . . to rid your very own body . . . of those nasty cancer cells . . .

You know . . . you know that your hair can be replaced . . . can be replaced . . . as your body gets new . . . thick hair . . . that can grow in its place . . .

And now . . . now I want you to know . . . that you have all the tools that you need to help you fight any possible side effects . . . of your medication and treatment . . . and because you are a fighter . . . , you can use them . . . You can use any of these whenever you wish . . .

Now sometimes . . . sometimes you may just feel like retreating . . . and going to your own special place . . . your very own special place . . . wherever you like to be . . . to be calm and relaxed . . . relaxed and calm . . . and that's fine . . . That is perfectly fine . . . and at these times, you can just relax . . . as you let the healing take place . . . in your very own special place . . . and wherever your body needs healing . . . You know that you can put your healing hand . . . and you can allow that part of your body to be healed . . . So allow your body to be healed . . . gently . . . slowly . . . easily . . . be healed . . . as you relax and let go of any worries . . . cares . . . or concerns . . .

And now . . . now if you have not already done so . . . , I want you to imagine yourself going to your very own special place right now . . . picture that scene . . . perhaps a beautiful day . . . You can hear the beautiful sounds . . . you can smell the aromas . . . or you maybe even able to touch this very own special place . . . whatever is good for you . . . Just enjoy your very own special place . . . Enjoy this very own special place . . .

I will leave you here for a short while . . . and when you next hear my voice . . . , I will bring you back . . . slowly gently back . . . with all the good feelings . . . that this special place brings to you . . .

Bring back . . .

# Relaxation for Brain Tumour

**Script . . .**

And as you relax deeper and deeper . . . deeper and deeper . . . , you can remember . . . you can remember that ever since the day you were born . . . , you have learned and experienced something in every day of your life . . . in every moment of your life . . . and all those experiences have been stored away . . . in the back of your mind . . . your very own subconscious mind . . . that has full access to all those images . . .

And as you drift away into your inner world . . . into that most inner part of yourself . . . that remembers all that you have experienced . . . and as you begin to pay more attention to all these inner thoughts and realities . . . , you are becoming more deeper relaxed . . . more deeply relaxed . . . You are remembering long forgotten memories . . . long forgotten delightful memories . . . inner feelings of safety an security . . . and the more you feel these feelings . . . , the deeper relaxed you feel . . .

You may find now . . . that your mind begins to wander . . . and it doesn't matter where your mind drifts . . . and as your mind drifts, you will notice the sound of my voice going with you . . . It will travel along with you . . . no matter where you are . . .

And now . . . now I would like you to know . . . that one of the nicest things about hypnosis is the trance-like state . . . and in that trance-like state . . . , you are capable of doing anything that you care to bring to mind . . . and in this wonderful relaxed state . . . , you can imagine yourself in your very own special place . . . and in this special place . . . , you can make changes within yourself . . . like allowing yourself to feel positive about the future . . . or using your very own body defences . . . to help in the healing process of your very own body . . .

You can use this healing process to help your very own immune system . . . to become stronger and stronger . . . stronger and stronger . . . to work alongside the treatments you are receiving . . . to move the healing process of your very own body . . . along . . . much more rapidly . . . smoothly . . . gently . . .

And now . . . now I want you to imagine the anti-bodies within you . . . Your anti bodies are the part of you . . . that fight off disease and illness . . . and I would like you to imagine these anti-bodies as tiny warrior soldiers . . .

And these soldiers are preparing to fight for you . . . to fight against the cancerous cells in your brain . . . You see these soldiers now . . . growing in numbers . . . And they now outnumber those cancer cells . . . by millions to one . . . growing stronger more and more . . . more and more . . . stronger . . . powerful . . . with each and every second . . .

I want you know to imagine these powerful soldiers . . . now making their way to the area of your discomfort . . . taking care of any other problems or discomforts along the way . . .

Now . . . now I would like you to imagine . . . in a way that is most beneficial to you . . . your warrior soldiers . . . attacking and destroying the cancerous cells . . . see them being destroyed powerfully . . . easily . . . and effectively . . . leaving all the other healthy cells untouched . . . You can take as long as you need to do this . . . and when you are finished . . . , you can let me know with a gentle nod of your head . . .

And now . . . now I would like you to imagine a tiny ball of light . . . at the site of where those cancerous cells used to be . . . Imagine this ball of light growing to the size of a golf ball . . . and from this light, you can feel a soothing warmth . . . a healing white light . . . and this healing white light continues to grow . . . to grow now the size of a tennis ball . . . and the warmth and healing now begins to spread throughout your brain . . . and as it becomes bigger and bigger . . . brighter and brighter . . . , it spreads down throughout your entire body . . .

And as the warmth spreads down . . . , this wonderful healing white light . . . brings feelings of well-being and comfort . . . that continue to spread throughout your entire body . . . and I want you to just enjoy those feelings of warmth and relaxation for a few more minutes . . .

Pause sixty seconds . . .

And now . . . now anytime in the future when you are at home . . . , you can continue to work with your warrior soldiers . . . and this healing light . . .

It is now time to come back to the room . . .

Bring slowly . . . gently . . . back . . .

# Pre-Surgery

**Script . . .**

And now . . . now very soon you will be having your pre-med . . . for your operation . . . before going to the theatre for the surgeons to work on healing your very own body . . . to heal your very own body . . .

Now . . . now I would like to prepare your mind . . . your very own subconscious mind . . . to accept . . . to accept willingly the help that you will receive . . . from all the doctors . . . the nurses . . . and they will instruct your body to heal and recover . . . far more quickly than would normally be possible . . .

And when the time comes . . . when the time comes to receive your anaesthesia . . . , you will be comfortably relaxed . . . and completely detached from what is happening . . .

And now . . . now even before the nurse numbs the back of your hand . . . ready to insert the needle that is connected to your very own drip . . . , your hand will feel like a soft piece of wood . . . that is floating on water . . .

And although there may be just a little bit of pressure in that area at first . . . , you won't feel any discomfort at all . . . as your very own mind is distracted in your very own special place . . . for you know that you are going to be in the most capable hands possible . . . because all those doctors and nurses . . . are the best in their field of work . . .

For you know . . . you know that they have all done years of training . . . and have performed many . . . many operations successfully on other patients . . . , who are now recovered . . . and are leading a healthy and happy life . . . far better than they ever thought possible to lead . . .

And it is because you trust them . . . just as you trust the sound of my voice . . . and you are fully prepared . . . and happy . . . about all that is going to happen . . .

And because . . . because in just a few hours . . . you will be on the road to recovery . . . , you will wonder why you did feel apprehensive . . . about any of the worries . . . concerns . . . that you did have . . .

So now . . . now concentrate on my voice more and more . . . more and more . . . and as you do so . . . you allow your mind to wander . . . to wander and explore all those wonderful images that flow into your very own imagination . . . for you are about to embark on a journey of discovery . . . to a special magical place . . .

And this . . . this magical special place . . . is so alive . . . with vibrant colours . . . and harmonious sounds . . . You feel calm and safe . . . safe and calm . . .

The scenery that you see is beautiful . . . and all around you . . . you sense a feeling of harmony . . . within yourself . . . and you allow yourself . . . to feel the warmth of the sun . . . the gentle warmth . . . penetrating every nerve and cell in your body . . . and every consciousness of your entire body is totally . . . completely . . . relaxed . . . and at peace . . .

Your mind and body are working in harmony together . . . together for the highest benefit for you . . . for everyone that is around you . . . and the rays of the sun . . . are full of healing love and energy . . . and you can feel this being transferred to your whole body . . .

And as you drift more and more into deeper relaxation . . . , you dream . . . You can dream of how it will be for you after your surgery . . . your operation . . . You see yourself healthy . . . your whole body functioning properly and normally . . . and you know that this is how you will feel when you arouse from this beautiful sleep-like state that you are in . . .

And now . . . now you see yourself carrying out ordinary . . . everyday tasks . . . with a completely new attitude of mind . . . because you now appreciate every aspect of your life . . . You have vitality . . . positive thoughts and feelings . . .

And every job that you do . . . even the most mundane jobs . . . seem so pleasurable for you . . . and as you focus your very own mind . . . on whatever it is you do . . . , you feel so good . . . You feel so wonderfully calm . . . relaxed and at peace . . . You feel so alive . . . happy . . . and you make the most of each and every moment of your wonderful life . . . your wonderful life ahead of you . . .

Now . . . now as you dream all your dreams . . . , you begin to feel more and more . . . more and more . . . the feeling of healing . . . health and vitality . . . Your whole body is breathing . . . is breathing the air . . . the life force . . . the prana . . . the chi . . . into your whole body . . . and as it does so . . . the purity of the oxygen that is being carried around your whole bloodstream . . . soothes and heals every cell in your body . . .

Now . . . now all the organs . . . cells . . . of your entire body . . . are working in perfect harmony . . . Your whole metabolism is tuning in with your very own body's individual needs . . .

Your digestive system now uses the food that you eat more effectively . . . and you now only eat the right amount of healthy . . . nutritious . . . food . . . that your body needs for its own healthy . . . way of being . . . You only desire the foods that are so good for you . . . and as you do so . . . , you allow yourself to adjust to your new and relaxed state . . . in perfect harmony with your mind and body . . .

And now . . . now your entire nervous system . . . begins to function . . . more effectively . . . and you feel a harmonious well-being flow throughout your whole body . . . your kidneys . . . your digestion system . . .

The blood supply to all your vital organs . . . such as your liver . . . your pancreas . . . your spleen . . . will nourish all your organs . . . as the chemistry in you and your body . . . becomes more balanced and stable . . .

Your brain waves are becoming more balanced . . . and a more peaceful and restful energy washes over you . . . and because of this, you will find you are sleeping more soundly and experiencing beautiful . . . wonderful dreams . . . and because of your biochemical and metabolic state . . . , your overall resistance to infections and diseases improves and your blood pressure is normal . . . as you go about your day-to-day activities . . . with a calm serenity and peace . . .

Your mind and body now . . . experience healing and health in a natural way . . . and as you look all around you at the beauty of nature . . . , you appreciate more and more . . . the quality of your life . . . and you feel as though you really are walking on air . . . happier and healthier than ever before . . . You see and feel such an immense improvement . . . on your whole being . . .

When you went into the theatre . . . , the lights shone down . . and the medical team . . . appeared like angels . . . sent down from heaven . . . to help you in your time of need . . . and your trust in that team was strengthened by the love that you felt . . . and the desire that you had . . . to recover . . . and regain . . . your state of health and vitality . . . Your mind was so calm . . . just as it is now . . .

And as you immerse yourself into a gentle hypnotic rest . . . , you see yourself on a magical and mystical journey . . . into the special place that you have created . . . ready to awaken after your rest . . . fully recovered and healed . . . and now . . . now you see a door in your special place . . . a white door . . . overgrown with moss and hanging leaves . . . but the door can open anytime you wish . . . into a beautiful cavern . . .

This cavern is a beautiful place . . . full of crystals . . . jade . . . sapphires . . . diamonds . . . and other precious stones and minerals . . . all hanging from the ceilings and walls of the cavern . . . and there is a beautiful blue light that reflects and shimmers . . . sparkling . . . alive with energy and love . . . and when you are ready to venture forward in, there you will experience a oneness with all creation . . . and all knowledge . . .

And . . . and as my voice fades . . . , you can allow yourself to explore . . . and you may even hear the sounds of nurses . . . doctors . . . from a distance . . . and as you do so . . . , any requests from those doctors . . . those nurses . . . will be beneficial for the future and well-being of yourself . . .

And as my voice fades more and more . . . , you will remain in this hypnotic state . . . all the way through surgery . . . and for a short time afterwards . . . while your body fully recovers . . .

Bring safely back . . .

# LIVING WITH CANCER: RELAXATION

**Script . . .**

And as you relax more and more . . . more and more . . . , your subconscious mind is open and receptive to suggestions that are given . . . allowing your imagination take you on a wonderful . . . magical journey . . . around your whole body . . . and you know what . . . ? Your body . . . your body will continue to look after you . . . for your whole life . . . and will continue to do so for a long time to come . . .

Do you know . . . do you know that the body has a remarkable ability to heal itself . . . ? Can you remember . . . how many times as a child . . . that you cut or bruised yourself . . . ? And do you remember how all those cells in your body . . . rushed to release any pain you were feeling . . . and healed your cuts and bruises . . . ? How remarkable that was . . . !

Now . . . now each cell in your body has a memory . . . which is how we build up our immunity from all childhood diseases and illnesses . . . and do you know that every muscle . . . every nerve . . . every gland in your body . . . is composed of little . . . tiny . . . cells . . . and those little . . . tiny . . . cells . . . hold every memory . . . hold on to every memory that you have . . . ?

And today . . . today . . . we . . . you . . . I . . . are going to gather up . . . and collect . . . all the memories . . . that you . . . that you need to fight that cancer . . . that does not belong to your body . . . and all those memories are going to help to produce perfect cells . . . to produce the perfect balance of living . . . healthy . . . cells . . . and cancer grows and occurs . . . when certain cells in your body . . . start to display uncontrolled growth . . . They then start to attack . . . destroy the living tissues in your body . . . , and those cells are the cells that we . . . I . . . you . . . are going to target during this hypnotic . . . trance-like state . . .

So now . . . now I want you to imagine . . . imagine yourself becoming smaller . . . and smaller . . . , and as you do so . . . , I want you to imagine . . . in front of you . . . a wet suit . . . the sort of wet suit that divers would use . . . going out into the sea . . .

And as you imagine that wet suit . . . laid out in front of you . . . , I invite you . . . to feel its texture . . . It is made of a soft form of rubber . . . and it feels very warm and comfortable against your skin . . . as you gently zip it up . . . feeling safe and warm . . . protected and safe . . .

And now . . . now you tie the belt bag around your waist . . . the bag is a sponge bag . . . and has a drawstring . . . which you tie together . . . and this bag is your very favourite colour . . . , and in this bag, I am going to invite you to put all those memory cells into . . .

But before you do . . . , I want you to look inside the bag . . . to notice that it is empty at the moment . . . and the inside of the bag . . . is padded . . . and safe . . . to protect all those important memory cells . . .

So now . . . now you have that bag tied to your waist . . . I would like you to see in front of you . . . your very own tool kitbag . . . and in this bag, you have all the tools you need during your journey ahead . . . including a pair of special goggles . . . which will help you to see and detect the malignant cells . . . in your body . . .

I know want you to tie this bag to the other side of your belt . . . on your wet suit . . . and you feel safe and protected . . . protected and safe . . . and when you are ready . . . , you imagine yourself diving into your very own body . . . You feel yourself entering your very own body . . . and you begin to swim around . . .

I want you know . . . to imagine how the inside of your body must look like to your cells . . . how huge those vital organs are . . . and those veins that carry your life force throughout your whole body . . . carrying the essential and vital nutrients . . . oxygen . . . to every cell in your body . . .

You notice your heart . . . beating gently and in time . . . You see your kidneys doing their daily work . . . flushing out those toxins . . . and all those cells that you see before your eyes . . . are your army . . . ready to deal with any invaders that may come your way . . . These cells recognise you . . . and they greet you warmly and gently . . . for they know that you are their leader . . . someone who will guide them into battle . . .

Now . . . now before we forward . . . to swim around your body . . . , I want to make sure that you feel safe and comfortable . . . comfortable and safe . . . and I want you to feel that you are protected as we swim around . . . You have your very own tool kit . . . on your waist that you can use any time that you wish . . .

And before you go . . . , I would like you to introduce yourself to all those cells that have come here today . . . to thank them . . . for all the good work that they are going to do for you . . . here today . . . this moment in time . . .

Ready now . . .

Let's begin . . .

OK . . . bring your attention back to my voice . . . Listen to my voice . . . Listen even more closely to my voice . . . We are now looking for all those healthy cells to form an army . . . to form an army that can destroy those invading cancer cells . . . You can notice this by seeing a fluorescent signal . . . that all the healthy cells give off . . .

So now . . . now you carefully remove the goggles from your bag . . . and you put them on . . . and you begin to swim around . . . you begin to swim around for the strongest . . . healthiest . . . cells that you can find . . . all the ones that give off the most powerful signals . . . and . . . and when you see them . . . , I would like you to invite them . . . to invite them in your journey ahead . . .

And . . . and these cells are friendly . . . and will be so happy . . . to join you . . . , so you invite them to come with you and place themselves in your soft . . . comfortable bag . . . on the side of your waist . . . eager to learn what you have in store for them . . . You will invite the strongest and healthiest cells you can find . . .

Now . . . now when your bag is full . . . , I invite you to swim up to the control room . . . the centre of all your being . . . and as you swim up to your very own control room . . . , there is a large table . . . and you place your bag on to that table . . . You open that bag . . . and you watch as all those healthy cells climb out of your bag . . . on to the table . . . They sit around that table . . . awaiting eagerly for their instructions . . . in what it is they can do to help you . . . in your conquest . . . in your mission . . . They will do whatever it takes to help you . . .

So now . . . now you explain to them in great detail . . . about the cancerous invaders that are invading your body . . . You tell them that they are the invaders that they have come here to destroy . . . Now . . . now you show them your tool kit . . . You show them your bag . . . and you allow them to choose whichever tools they feel that they would need . . . to be the most useful in their battle ahead . . .

And each one of these tools . . . contains a magic bullet . . . and these bullets can only kill and destroy malignant cells . . . and I want you to know . . . to know that the healthier ones will always be protected . . . from the effects of those magic bullets . . .

Do you know . . . do you know that your healthy cells have a unique memory . . . and they hold within them the ability to search out . . . and detect the cancerous cells, . . . and as they do so, they will have you to guide and lead them along the way . . . ?

And now . . . now you watch as one by one . . . all those healthy cells . . . move quickly back into the soft and protected bag . . . carrying all the tools and magic bullets along with them . . . You now put the bags back on to your belt . . . and strap it up tightly . . . and now . . . now you prepare yourself for your journey ahead . . . You are still wearing your special goggles . . . and you know exactly where it is you need to go . . .

And as you swim . . . , all those malignant cells have a easily recognised signal . . . and they are so easy to detect . . . and, within seconds, you are there . . . You are there in the part of the body where those malignant cells . . . sit and reside . . . And now . . . now you open your bag . . . and all those healthy cells and their tools and magic bullets . . . climb and swim out . . . awaiting for your orders when to attack . . . Your healthy cells swim to a safe place . . . from where they will commence their attack . . . and their elimination of cancerous cells . . .

They instantly recognise the invaders and you know that it is safe to return to the outside world . . . and to allow the battle to take place . . . , so now . . . say goodbye . . . for now . . . to the cells in your body . . . and return to the outside world . . . and as you do so . . . , you remove your wet suit and you begin to forget about this journey now . . .

And as you do so . . . , you allow your subconscious mind to remind those cells of their task . . . and your subconscious mind will continue to do this constantly . . . until all those malignant cells are destroyed . . . and harmony is restored . . . , balance is restored again . . .

These suggestions are firmly embedded in your subconscious mind . . . and they grow stronger and stronger . . . day by day . . . They grow stronger by the day . . . stronger by the hour . . . stronger by the minute . . . stronger and stronger . . . stronger and stronger with every passing second . . .

And now . . . in a moment, I am going to count down from ten to one . . . and when I reach one . . . , you will be wide awake . . . feeling so wonderfully alive . . . and so ready to allow all those suggestions . . . those magic bullets . . . to work for you . . .

Bring back . . . safely and gently . . .

Welcome back . . .

# Hypnosis and the Relief of Pain

Pain is a growing concern for many who have cancer and terminal illness. It is very important to stress that pain, either in an acute or chronic form (due to surgery or resulting from the growth of tumours in some parts of the body), that although hypnotic pain control can be very useful in these situations; it must be used carefully, and not to hide or mask pain that is caused by the ongoing progression of the disease.

Therefore, it is very important that any help offered to a patient, either by a trained hypnotherapist or family member, always has written medical consent to treat clients with pain control and to fully understand the ethical implications.

## So what is pain?

Pain is defined by the International Association for the Study of Pain as 'an unpleasant sensory and emotional experience associated with actual or potential tissue damage or described in terms of such damage'.

All medications which are used to block pain are called analgesics, and the term *hypnoanalgesia* is used in hypnotherapy for using an analgesic to control pain.

Many of us are more afraid of pain than we are of dying, and pain instils fear into us because along with the sensory experiences it creates, there are feelings of vulnerability and a loss of control.

In the very early years of the human race, people regarded pain as the work of demons and believing that it was of the work of sorcerers, shamans, and priests. They used many methods to control pain, including the use of medicinal herbs, ceremonies, rituals, and journeying to the other worlds (often known as soul retrieval). Pain and death at this time was often regarded as much more of a part of life, and the methods that used and enjoyed in pain relief were not always the same as orthodox medicine used today.

There was an idea that the nervous system had a part to play in the perception of pain and was originally developed by the Greeks and the Romans, and it was not until the fourteen hundreds onwards that these theories started to gain evidential support. Leonardo da Vinci was the first person who came to the conclusion that the brain played a central role in the perception of sensations. He also proposed and developed that the concept of the spinal cord played a big part in the process.

Next was the philosopher, Descartes, and he was responsible for what he termed the 'pain pathway', describing how 'particles of fire' in contact with the feet travelled to the brain.

It wasn't until the nineteenth century that science became more as we know it is today, and this is when it started to make waves in the relief of pain. With the finding of cocaine, codeine, and opium came the big advances in using drugs as a relief of pain. It was these major advances that led to the discovery of aspirin and the development of local and general anaesthetics.

Pain is used by the body as a warning signal that all is not right within our physical body and also covers up our emotional states and selves, often masking the pain with a physical pain within the body.

It is very much worth pointing out that our body reflects our mind, and it is our mind's way of asking for help.

Without the ability to feel pain, we would be in very serious trouble, as we would continue to damage tissue and ignore the symptoms of illness, which would eventually cause demise in the body.

How is all this relevant to treating and helping someone with cancer and in hospice and palliative care? We need to know in hypnotherapy the levels of pain that the patient is in, and in its chronic form, it can deeply affect our mobility as well as our state of mental and emotional health. Added to this is the difficulty with which some people seem to have different pain thresholds, which makes it harder for those with a higher threshold to understand the effect that pain has on others.

Pain can be divided into two types. They are as follows:

- **Acute pain**—the majority of these concern pain that results from disease, inflammation, or injury. It will generally come on suddenly and be accompanied by anxiety or emotional distress. It is treatable and is defined by the fact that it will have an ending and will decrease as the body begins to heal itself. In some cases, it will move on to chronic pain.
- **Chronic pain**—this type of pain persists over a longer period of time and is often made worse by the environment that the person is living in and their psychological state. Chronic pain is very often resistant to orthodox medical treatments.

Pain can be felt in a variety of ways, for example, a burning sensation, a sharp prick, an ache, or a tingling sensation. The start of the experience is that receptors on the skin cause a sequence of signals that travel to the spinal cord. The spinal cord is a very effective pathway where the signal can be blocked, enhanced, or even modified before it reaches the brain. Once in the brain, the pain signals to the thalamus, before going on down to the cortex (which is the thinking part of the brain). The thalamus also plays a part in relaying messages between the brain and various areas of the body as well as storing images of the body. This process explains the phenomena of amputees who still experience pain in the missing limb. The sensation of pain is produced by a complicated process that involves some of the body's neurotransmitters (which are chemical messengers that pass signals from one nerve cell to another). Some of these are responsible for severe pain and others are responsible for milder pain sensations.

Hypnosis can be used to help in both types of pain, although acute pain is often better helped by the patient learning or having learnt self-hypnosis.

Chronic pain (by its definition) can be helped by hypnosis both by a practitioner and by the person using self-hypnosis.

At the time of writing this book, it is not fully understood how hypnosis works in the treatment of pain, but the fact remains that hypnosis does work for some people. Hypnosis is generally used to control and contain the amount of pain that a person can stand, and the use of relaxation techniques seems to assist in a person's ability to deal with the pain, and the reduction of anxiety helps further.

Hypnosis may also be very useful with the effect it may have on some of the chemicals that are working within the nervous system and the effect that certain impulses within the body are slowed down.

The main factors that affect our response to pain are hormones, psychology, culture, and the environment. It is also quite possible that the way that pain and illnesses were approached when we were young and growing up does have an affect with how we deal with pain later on in our lives.

There is a general consensus in the field of science and medicine that pain affects men and women differently and that research supports the ongoing belief that there is a higher number of women that seek help from their GP regarding their pain than men. Women, in general, will seek help much sooner, will seek better coping strategies, and are also less likely to allow pain to control their everyday lives than men. It is also suggested that women will feel pain at a lower threshold than that of men.

There is an interesting fact that stimulating the sense of smell in women with pleasant odours has the effect of reducing the problems caused by pain, but this only seems to work in general for women.

Another example of the ways that pain affects women and men in different ways is in the use if some painkilling drugs. Morphine, for instance, tends to work better for men than it does for women, while it does seem possible that the onset of pain comes quickly for women, but they then can tolerate pain much more than men.

## Natural painkillers

There is a strong belief that the most effective methods of pain relief are found and lie within our own body. These are endorphin and enkephalin.

The term *endorphin* means *morphine from within*, and these chemicals can bind to the receptors on nerve cells to provide relief from pain in the brain. It is this process that prevents us from feeling pain when we receive a severe injury, gives us the high that we get from intense exercise, as well as the pain relief we obtain from acupuncture and chiropractic work. The 'endorphin high' has been used to explain why so many people enjoy the experience of being tattooed and why some continue to tattoo their entire bodies.

The process of discovering endorphins and their effects has evolved over the years. In the mid-sixties, the connection was made by discovering the analgesic effect of a pituitary hormone, and also when scientists in America were trying to work out the reason that opium has the effects it does on the human system, and when doing so, they found the 'opiate' receptors in the brain. Research continued, and it was found that the receptors seemed to be mainly in the areas that deal with the integration and perception of pain and emotions. If a person is in pain, then the presence of 'opiates' will diminish the discomfort, and if there is no significant pain present, then the result of the presence of 'opiates' will be to create a feeling of euphoria.

It wasn't until 1975 that the substances that we refer to as endorphins were isolated in the brain by scientists. Endorphins can either instigate the fight or flight response, or even the idea of a 'reward system', and this is why some people seem to be addicted to their production.

Neurotransmitters are defined as substances and chemical messengers that transport messages through the network of nerve cells, and these can be compared to the action of endorphins as modulators. They modulate rather than pass on the feelings of pain and pleasure that we experience. Endorphins act by inhibiting the nerves in the frontal lobe of the brain, which results in the reduction of the feelings of pain, by allowing a flood of dopamine (neurotransmitter) that will result in the sensations of euphoria.

The transmission of the pain impulse to the brain seems to be managed by a substance known as 'substance P', and the actions of endorphins may prevent the release of this substance, which will reduce our sensitivity to pain.

The placebo effect that is seen in some people when they experience positive side effects from being given an 'inert' pill can be attributed to our very own painkillers in our body, as we emotionally feel 'good' about being given a pill that we are led to believe will make us better.

From all this, we can see that our bodies are able to deal with pain to some extent and degree and that people's ability to deal with pain will differ from person to person and the extent of pain. Another large impact on the effect in the way we experience pain is the amount of fear and anxiety that we can associate with this and how it makes us feel.

Fear adds to the pain experience, and stress and anxiety will make it worse. When treating people for pain and physical illnesses, it is of upmost importance to bear all the facts in mind and to be aware of all these implications. The reduction of fear will reduce anxiety and will make the pain or illness easier to cope with.

## Acute pain

Acute pain is either due to trauma or the presence of a chronic condition. The way we experience pain is generally seen as being subjective, and the effective assessment of pain is best done by those experiencing it. This is because the way in which we feel pain is not just a physical phenomena but also an environmental and psychological one as well. The sensory perception of acute pain can also be influenced by past experience and any emotions that are present.

The experience of acute pain may be a useful indication to the individual to the extent of which the pain is affecting the illness or any life-threatening illness. The ability to control pain in serious illnesses is a huge relief to the sufferer.

Another type of pain, which is often used, is the term *iatrogenic pain*, which refers to the pain we experience and the fear we are going to experience when a medical procedure is carried out (there is pain, but it is an aid to the healing process).

Fear and anticipation of any given pain causes as much difficulty as the pain does itself, and, in fact, the fear that we feel in those situations is warranted, as the subconscious receives the message that the body is experiencing another trauma.

It is very much an important note to mention here in this chapter on 'pain relief' that it is essential that you never treat anyone with acute pain who has not been through the appropriate diagnostic procedures with a qualified medical doctor, and if this is the case, then you should always obtain written permission from a doctor or consultant.

*It should also be remembered that the use of hypnotherapy should be part of an effective and comprehensive treatment plan and not as a stand-alone treatment, and it should never be used to mask symptoms that may well be developing.*

Hypnosis has been used for many centuries, but to this day, it is still not sure how it works. There are many methods that can be used, and the use of any of these methods should be client-led. Hypnosis can be used to assist people to cope with any future acute pain, before an anticipated trauma, for relaxation and coping strategies after the trauma of an operation and so on. It can also be used in a mixture of these ways to assist those with a diagnosis of terminal illness, which can give the person a feeling of regaining some control over the situation, which will, in turn, reduce anxiety.

Although *cancer* is still a word that strikes terror into the hearts of many people, there are many types of cancer that are now treatable, and it is common knowledge that the treatment is often unpleasant and painful. This can be in either an acute or chronic form due to surgery or even pain from the growth of tumours in some parts of the body. Hypnotic pain control can be very useful in such situations, but you must always be careful not to mask any pain caused by a progression of the disease that should be noted and treated further.

When people are diagnosed with terminal illness, or when they are coming to the end of their life, they may have a certain amount of time before they die to reflect on their life and the things that they would like to do, if possible, before their time comes. The idea of therapeutic intervention at this time can bring a deeper acceptance and a sense of peace to all those around them.

In the present time of diagnosis, there does not seem to be the same policy of doctors giving an exact life expectancy. As you might be aware by now, in the reading of this book, the power of suggestion is very, very strong and can have an effect of causing someone to give up and die when they have been told that they are going to. This can often go the other way with someone with a rebellious personality who wish to prove the doctors wrong.

With this in mind, it is easier to see how using the power of suggestion using hypnotherapy can have a great benefit in the relieving of pain in those with cancer and terminal illness. By the assisting of people with the reduction of pain levels can make their last days much better for them and their family ensuring that they are not mentally affected by the strong painkilling drugs that are given at this time. This can make the surviving relatives and friends' grief process easier to go through, as they are very often able to communicate with the person who is dying much closer to the end. Learning relaxation techniques can also be of great value as the brain is given time off from the constant and relentless pressure of the knowledge that a person is living with a terminal illness.

## A word about hypnotic techniques

There are many types of scripts that are and can be written in the appropriate cases of acute and chronic pain, and the only true effective approach is to work on someone on an individual basis, being fully aware of the issues that the patient has. It is highly important to remember that the perception of pain is very much individual and that not everyone is able to be helped.

The best way to start is by helping someone to relax both their body and their mind, and in doing so, the perception of pain can be reduced or erased when total relaxation is achieved. We need to achieve the client in realising the times when their body and mind is signalling that they are having trouble dealing with stress around the situation that they are facing. This will involve (by suggestion) the acceptance of their situation and the total recognition of the things that they need to change in order to have the best quality of life they have left.

It is also essential that the patient has the ability to prepare for pain; this enables pain control to be easier than if pain hits a person unawares, and practice is of the upmost importance here. Pain cause us to tense up due to the fear that it instils in us, and if we are tense, then it makes it that much more difficult to employ and use pain reduction strategies. Being aware of the possibility of pain can prevent a build-up of tension in the mind and body.

## Using glove anaesthesia

One of the most widely used and accepted ways of treating pain is the use of 'glove anaesthesia' in hypnosis.

Glove anaesthesia can be created in a variety of ways, which involves hot or cold. As long as a person can achieve a medium state of hypnosis, they should be able to experience some positive results with this method. But you should always make sure that this method is the right one for the patient.

A post-hypnotic trigger using this method is installed by suggesting that the patient will experience glove analgesia when they think or say an appropriate phrasing such as 'I feel my hand going numb'. The hand is the place on the part of the body that is causing the pain, which then transfers the numbness to the given area. This method does take some practice on both parts and can be very effective.

There are many ways to achieve this numb feeling in the hand, and they include as follows:

- Imagining a nerve block injection
- Imagining sensations of heat (for example, the sun)
- Imagining a bowl of ice
- Imagining putting on a glove that causes numbness (very good for imaginative clients)
- The application of a safe numbing substance

## Suggestion work around endorphin production

It is possible to increase the production of endorphins in the body by using the power of suggestion. The suggestions can involve images of the brain producing these chemicals and then bathing the affected area of pain in them, or you could imagine the messengers produced by the brain, sending powerful messages to reduce the amount or sensation of pain. Another way of achieving this is to introduce the concept of visiting the part of the brain that is host to pain control (using the image of a control board or dial, the patient can adjust the switches or dial that are producing the endorphins to increase production and send the chemicals to the offending area of the body).

Another approach could be that as the brain is responsible for the prevention of the pain, it could be suggested that the brain is in some way prevented from picking up these signals, or it may seem to be engaged on another matter, which will distract from receiving the signals that are creating the pain.

*It is of the upmost importance that these suggestions are left in the control of the patient. The perception of pain should never be turned off for an unspecified amount of time, and the suggestions should only be used to control pain when the actual source of the pain is completely understood.*

The range and scope of the useful suggestion can be as varied as both the patient and the hypnotherapist are concerned, and it is always best the treatment is client-led. They need to be in control of the pain, and they themselves know their own body far better than anybody else.

*It is worth remembering that in controlling pain, we can control our own anxiety over our condition, and we will then be able to see things more clearly in our condition and course of treatment.*

## A note for the future

Those who are managing such chronic conditions and acute pain in cancer, hospice, and palliative care are now much more open to using complementary therapies such as hypnosis. There is a growth in this area and can only be good for the benefit and welfare of the patient to have access to hypnotherapy and the relief of pain.

There is a certain amount of perception that orthodox medicine works for everything and that people are moving away from such ideas, realising that there such few therapies or medications that provide a cure—all for any condition. In doing so, this enables the power to be given back to the person living with the condition and enables them to feel more in control of the process that they are going through.

*This doesn't change the fact that they may shortly be dying, but it does give them the power to say how they die and have a choice in doing so. We all should be allowed to have that right and be given the freedom to do so without the judgement of others.*

*After all, it is our life and not anybody else's*

## Glove Anaesthesia and Relaxation

### Script . . .

And now . . . now as you relax more and more . . . , I want you to imagine that you are in a beautiful wooden chalet high up in the mountains . . . and in your very own wooden chalet, you have a roaring . . . blazing open log fire . . . There are bundles of logs all tied up together . . . all laying beside the side of the fire . . . You look around your wooden chalet and you notice a large . . . wooden . . . heavy oak table . . . and on this table are cups . . . glasses . . . and a lovely fruit bowl . . . filled up . . . right to the top . . . with fresh fruit . . . apples . . . oranges . . . grapes . . . bananas . . . pears . . .

And outside . . . outside your warm lovely wooden chalet . . . , it is a crisp . . . cold, and snowy day . . . The snow is lying on the ground like a thick carpet . . . and there is a snowman in the garden . . . with eyes and a nose . . . with a lovely smile . . . looking back at you . . . and inside . . . inside the fire is crackling . . . and the flames are dancing . . . giving off a warm orange . . . in colour . . . glow . . . and this fire is a fire that you just want to kneel in front off . . . and feel the glowing embers of the fire . . . and in your hand is a lovely cup of hot chocolate . . . warming the insides of you . . . feeling warm and content . . . content and warm . . .

The whole chalet is so very warm and comfortable . . . and in the background is your favourite music playing on the radio . . . the sounds gently vibrating in the air . . . You look further around, and you notice a window in the corner of the room . . . You take a short walk over to the window . . . and you take a look outside . . . The window is playing host to the most wonderful view that you can imagine . . . outside . . . as the snowflakes gently come down from the sky . . . resting on the ground below . . . , and you watch as each snowflake in succession . . . gathers momentum on the window ledge . . . landing softly . . . and light as a feather . . . You look around the view outside . . . totally engrossed in the view . . . just watching and waiting for each snowflake to fall and settle . . .

And gradually below you . . . the ground becomes adorned with new . . . soft . . . white . . . blankets of snow . . . There are no footprints around . . . and you watch closely as snow settles on the trees . . . and the distant mountain range . . . seems so far away . . . the sky becoming darker and darker . . . heavier and heavier . . . with each and every moment . . .

It is so lovely and warm in here . . . and the fire is now crackling and blazing higher and higher . . . and as you look outside the window once more . . . the snow is piling up high . . . on the window sill . . . obscuring your vision . . . , and you light a lamp to help you see . . . beyond the blanket of snow . . . and before it gets too dark . . . , you decide that you would like to go outside . . . into the snow . . . and as you do, you imagine the first snows of winter . . . from childhood days long ago . . .

You eagerly put on your coat . . . hat . . . gloves . . . scarf . . . and you gently begin to open the door . . . The door is stiff and creaky . . . and you push a little harder . . . and the door opens slowly . . . allowing the cold . . . fresh . . . air . . . to come in . . . You step outside into the snow . . . and you feel your feet sinking . . . gently into the soft snow underneath . . .

And now . . . now I invite you to take off your glove on your right hand . . . and you pick up a handful of fresh . . . soft . . . snow . . . You feel your fingers as they begin to shape and mould the snow . . . into a snowball . . . that is hard and crisp to touch . . . and soon . . . soon, the palm of your hand on your right hand begins to go numb . . . The fingers on your right hand now also begin to go numb . . . and then . . . then your thumb starts to become tingly . . . cold . . . and then also becoming numb . . . Your hand . . . fingers . . . thumb . . . are cold and tingling . . . as the cold from the snow penetrates the skin of your hand . . .

Now . . . now your whole right hand is becoming numb from the icy cold snow . . . cold and numb . . . numb and cold . . . so icy cold that there is no feeling in your right hand any more . . .

Can you feel that now . . . your hands so cold and numb . . . ? That's good . . . Now I would like you to think of a place in your body . . . a place in your body where the discomfort was . . . and as you do so . . . you gently lift your right arm . . . and place it over the area where you know needs healing . . . Good . . . very good . . . You now place that cold . . . numb . . . right hand . . . on the part of you that is in need of healing . . . and rest it there . . . and as you rest it there . . . , you feel the snow beginning to melt . . . just a little . . . and the ice . . . cold . . . water . . . dripping on to your wrist . . .

You now begin to notice how that numbness . . . begins to transfer from that icy cold hand . . . to the part of you where the discomfort was . . . and as that area of your body becomes cold and numb . . . tingly . . . icy cold . . . , you notice that the numbness transfers to that area . . . and as it does so . . . it melts and dissolves away any discomfort . . . easing it gently away . . . and as that part of your body begins to heal itself . . . , you notice your right hand beginning to return back to normal . . .

And as your hand returns to normal . . . , you are aware that you can keep that numbness there . . . in the part of the body . . . that was in need of so much comfort . . . You now notice how the discomfort has eased away . . . gently melted and drained away . . . and all you can feel is the numb feeling there . . . in the area of the body that was in so much need for comfort . . . You have a very comfortable feeling inside you now . . . a very calm feeling . . . and you know what . . . ? You can keep that calm . . . comfortable feeling there . . . for as long as you want . . . and need to . . .

So you know now how to create anaesthesia in your body . . . any part of your body . . . and you find that you can do it so easily . . . and effortlessly . . . simply by taking three . . . big . . . deep . . . breaths . . . And counting the numbers down from ten to one . . . and with each and every descending number . . . , you will take yourself . . . deeper and deeper . . . deeper and deeper . . . into self-hypnosis . . . until . . . until you reach the number one . . . and are back at your wooden mountain cabin . . . where you allow your hand to become numb and cold . . .

And when your hand is numb and cold . . . , you will find that you will be easily able to transfer that numbness . . . to the part of your body . . . that is in need of healing . . . and you will be able to have that calm and comfortable feeling . . . for as long as you wish . . .

Bring safely . . . gently back . . .

# Writing Your Own Hypnosis Scripts

*Writing your very own hypnotherapy scripts is the best way to give the person that you are treating the best possible chance of success. This enables you to personalise the treatment plan, making sure that you have understood the needs of the patient.*

## The role of the subconscious

The conscious and subconscious are two separate parts of our mind. The conscious part of the mind is responsible for dealing with experiences that are occurring in the present, while the subconscious mind is the 'database' where we hold all our learning and experience. It also holds the keys to all our automatic reflexes and safety mechanisms in our bodily functions and movements.

Did you know?

- The subconscious will nearly always win over the conscious mind
- The subconscious role is primarily responsible for our survival
- The subconscious stores all the information that it is given
- The subconscious works in black and white; there are no grey areas
- The subconscious takes up ten-elevenths of the total mind
- The subconscious is responsible for all our involuntary physical processes (as well as our flight or fight mode)
- The subconscious cannot deal with any negative actions
- You can change any messages that our subconscious stores, as long as any new messages are of benefit for us

- The subconscious responds with instinct
- The subconscious is programmed to continually seek out and find more and more information
- The subconscious responds to symbols
- The subconscious works on the principle of least effort
- The subconscious needs repetition for longer projects

We are born with our subconscious functioning for our survival instincts, and it is only when the conscious mind develops later that any new messages to the subconscious allows us to experience them. Which means that as we gain more experiences, our very own powerful subconscious mind has a larger amount of experiences to store and work with. As it works with these messages, it creates our very own belief system.

The conscious mind has the ability to be critical of any suggestions made and will compare any possible actions. The subconscious will be in favour of the best action to take to ensure our survival instinct. It will aim to reduce our anxieties and worries in the quickest way possible.

Now between these two parts of the mind is something known as the 'conscious critical faculty' or CCF, which can be seen as a filter between the conscious and the subconscious mind. The CCF enables us to compare a new situation with our own belief system. In doing so, the conscious mind can assess if the subconscious mind is ready to deal with a situation or if indeed it is a new one.

*Hypnosis can be defined as a natural state of consciousness in which the conscious critical faculty is bypassed and an acceptable selective thinking process is established.*

The CCF can be suspended and can be viewed as a simple way of bypassing the evaluating, reasoning, judging part of our mind. The subconscious mind cannot be reasoning—this is the job of the conscious mind—the conscious mind can only reason with any information that is stored and housed from experience in the subconscious mind.

It is essential, therefore, that for the success in hypnosis to take place, the CCF is bypassed, and in doing so, some people will go into a deeper state of trance than others. The depth of trance can affect the outcome of the hypnotherapy session.

## What are the signs of hypnosis and trance-like state?

In understanding the signs of hypnosis, it is very evident that we may well all experience different ways. No one person is likely to be able to identify with all in the list that follows, but as a word of note, the vast majority of people can be hypnotised (with the exception of some very young children and those with severe psychiatric issues). There are observable and non-observable signs of hypnosis, and these can act as a guideline in assessing that the person you are treating has reached an acceptable state to bypass their CCF.

## Observable signs of hypnosis

- Swallowing—this is a relaxation response
- Eyelids fluttering
- Breathing becoming slower due to relaxation
- The body visually relaxing
- Reddening of the face
- Rapid eye movement
- An emotional response such as crying or laughing

The list is not exhaustive, and it is worth noting that hypnosis is completely normal and may well help to reduce any inhibitions that are stopping you from developing yourself as a person.

## Non-observable signs of hypnosis

- Tingling in feet, hands, legs, or arms
- Feelings of a change in weight—some people will experience feelings of heaviness and others of lightness. Some may even feel as if they are floating or sinking
- Heart rate slow down
- A feeling of time distortion—you may well feel like you have been in hypnosis for a lot less time than is actually the case
- Increased suggestibility—during hypnosis, people are more likely to accept beneficial changes due to the fact the CCF is bypassed, as long as the suggestions fit into their own moral codes (remember that you cannot be made to do anything that you wouldn't normally want to do anyway)
- There may be an internalised emotional response

The list above is not exhaustive, but a good indicator that the person who has been hypnotised is that they may well take awhile to return completely to full awareness.

## Depths of trance

The trance-like state is both dependent on both the person having hypnosis and the therapist. There are ways to assist the person to go into a deeper level of trance if needed to, but, ultimately, this will depend on the person itself. The best way to achieve a deeper level of trance is to personalise the scripts, and we will be looking at this further in this part of the book. It is remembering that many people will need a little practice before they reach the deepest state they can achieve and the building of rapport is vital to the outcome of hypnotherapy.

There are five main depths of trance, and they are as follows:

- **Mild state**—a person may well report to be at peace with themselves and, in some cases, aches and pains that they have been experiencing may well disappear. The eyelids may well flutter, and the eyes will remain shut, although there may well be an inclination towards sleep, the person will be aware what is going on externally. In this state, a good deal of suggestion work can be done, and people will often be able to achieve a deeper state in following sessions when rapport and anxiety have been increased and reduced.
- **Light state**—this state is achieved by the majority of people and is a good place for relaxation along with the focusing on issues that the person is here to work on. There will be a complete mental and physical relaxation. On occasions, the person may well be unable to open his or her eyes and sometimes will report that he or she also couldn't move his or her arms, legs, and so on. Breathing is slow and regular, and there is some feeling of mental detachment, although some will report that they really did not feel as though they had been hypnotised as they could hear all that was said!
- **Medium state**—this is the same state as above but also the possible ability of partial amnesia (loss of memory). The person will reorientate with feelings that something has happened but are unable to say what suggestions were made. Again analgesia (relief of pain) can also be experienced at this stage.

- **Somnambulism**—this is a very deep trance-like state in which the person can open his or her eyes and walk and talk under hypnosis. If his or her eyes are open, he or she will have a fixed stare. In this state, amnesia may be loosened, allowing for a definite recall of lost or repressed memories.
- **Esdaile or coma state**—it is possible to go into this state spontaneously. James Esdaile (a physician working in India), during the mid-1800s, induced trance-like states in his patients before anaesthesia was discovered and used in surgical operations. Esdaile used mesmeric hand movements and arm motions but now more modern techniques are used. In the 1800s, about 50 per cent of those having surgery did not survive, but Esdaile had a success rate of 80 per cent. Unfortunately, on Esdaile's return to England, people could not replicate his rate of success and eventually everyone lost faith in his abilities, and his career was lost and destroyed.

It wasn't until, a hundred years later, that a hypnotherapist called Dave Elman came across the hypnotic coma state which he found to be very similar (if not the same as) to the Esdaile trance-like state. Elman went on to use and teach this state, and its ability to reduce pain made it very popular.

People in this state are very often unwilling to come back, and if a person does go into this state, then it is important that you stay calm; they may well look grey and their breathing may be barely noticeable. You can return someone from this state by normal counting methods (using them with more forcefulness and volume than normal) or you can wait until the person returns naturally.

## The use of waking hypnosis

Suggestion work is not just a tool used during the hypnosis part of a therapy but also when you are talking to someone in a conscious state.

*Waking hypnosis is defined as 'the suggestions that are given to a person in a certain manner while they are in a normal state of consciousness, and they achieve a hypnotic effect without the use of a relaxed state'.*

The idea surrounding this is to allow the person to establish 'selective thinking'. Hypnosis is very successful when the person is totally focused on one thing only and by using the right words and body language, you can bypass the CCF. When doing so, it enables the person to accept any beneficial suggestions in a conscious state. Although this is not as effective as 'hypnosis', it does allow the treatment plan to proceed in a productive way. The reason why this works so effectively is that the person does not realise that you are using the technique, and they will suspend their critical judgement filter and any suggestions will begin to assist in allowing healing to begin.

## Facts about suspending the CCF

- In suspending the CCF, always retain good eye contact.
- In suspending the CCF, always talk in a sincere and caring way.
- Always focus on the benefits that the person will experience when they reach their goal in hypnosis.
- Always have a special chair for them in the hypnotic session.
- Use the word 'you' more often than 'I' and 'me', this will allow the person to realise that you are concentrating on them.
- After the hypnotic session ends, people are still more suggestible for at least another thirty to forty-five minutes, so repetition of the positive suggestions made will enhance their progress.
- If you look directly in the person's eyes, you will cause the CCF to be bypassed, as this makes many of us feel slightly uncomfortable.

## Suggestion work

When writing scripts, the formation of suggestions is very important for the overall success rate of hypnotherapy. The important thing to remember is that when you are writing your suggestions for scripts is that you are talking to the subconscious mind.

*When writing suggestions in your scripts, it is necessary to repeat suggestions in order for them to permanently replace the previous detrimental ones and aid in the healing process. Repeating suggestions is the best way to obtain the desired outcome for the person concerned.*

In writing scripts, it is advisable to:

- Avoid impossibilities—the best approach is to break down the therapy into achievable goals and work from there. This will increase the person's confidence as smaller goals are more achievable. You can then move on to higher goals.

- Do not use clichés—this can be detrimental to suggestion work. For example, words have different meanings, and the subconscious is very literal in accepting those suggestions. For example, weather has many different meanings.
- Using the correct timelines—make sure the suggestions are covering exactly what you want the outcome to be, for example, 'each and every day you are feeling better and better' is different from 'from this moment forward you are feeling better and better'.
- Positive suggestions—the very best hypnotic scripts are those that are totally positive and realistic. Please *bear in mind that when working with those with a terminal illness, in a hospice or receiving palliative care, to always be honest; they will respect you more; they deserve to be treated with respect, honesty, and dignity.* The subconscious is not very good with negatives and does not recognise the words such as 'can't' or 'won't'.

To summarise suggestions, they should be:

- Specific to the person's goal and outcome
- Literal in meaning
- Positive
- Avoiding unclear wordings
- Always use all the senses to improve and open up the resistance of the person's experiences

*Suggestion work should always be positive, positive, positive. The power of the mind is not to be underestimated.*

## The initial consultation and building rapport

The initial consultation is a very important part of the hypnotherapy session; it is where all the intended work to be done on the person is outlined and where a treatment plan can be put in place. It is imperative that all the skills needed to treat them are in place and there are not any ethical reasons why the treatment cannot go ahead.

It is where all the facts can be gathered and is where all the information about the person's health and current medication can be assessed.

*Always, always only work with the permission of the relevant people in the primary care of the person that you are intending to treat; it is for both their and your benefit.*

During the initial consultation, it gives a great idea on whether you both are compatible to continue working together and is a great way of building up rapport.

Rapport is a skill referring to the way in which we communicate, and communication is shown in the following ways:

- 55 per cent body language
- 38 per cent tone of voice
- 7 per cent content

When building rapport, first impressions are very important to build a good relationship. The person you will be treating will make various assumptions about you using their deductive logic, which is based on your appearance, your speech pattern, and your body language, and the same is true when you are meeting them for the first time.

*You need to bear in mind that if you are of a different personality type to themselves, they may well not respond to you as well as if you were to behave in a way that is similar to them.*

In order to build up rapport, the client needs to know that you are both listening and attending to them and their behaviour. This can be conveyed to them in different ways, using our own behaviour, body language, posture, and speech. Also it needs to be taken into account their own behaviour patterns.

There are attending and non-attending behaviours:

Attending behaviours

- Maintaining eye contact without a fixed stare
- Sitting next to the person or side on to them without placing a barrier in between
- Leaning slightly towards the person, although leaning too far will make them feel uncomfortable
- Adopting an 'open posture'
- Using encouraging responses such as smiling and nodding when appropriate

Non-attending behaviours

- Looking away from the client, around the room or down in front of them
- Fidgeting with ant objects that you may be holding
- Yawning
- Doodling
- Using a desk as a protective barrier
- Looking at your watch
- Closing your eyes
- Sitting too far away
- Adopting a closed posture

*Be aware how your behaviour comes across to the other person and also be aware of how you would feel if things were the other way around.*

## Empathy and sympathy

*When treating someone, it is very important to employ empathy and not sympathy.*

Being sympathetic is being able to feel what a situation is like for them and offering them pity and compassion. This approach does not lead them out of the situation that they are in but may, in turn, assist them to stay in the detrimental position that they are in.

When employing empathy, we enter into the feelings and the situation of the other person, but we do not 'jump in and join them'. The focus is on looking for a solution and helping them to choose the one that will suit them the most.

## Paraphrasing

Paraphrasing is about putting the person's words into our own words. It is done in a fewer amount of words than the person's own story. It is focusing on the facts rather than the emotions. When you have all the facts from the person, it cuts out the emotional content that people use in conversation when they are relating to a particularly difficult stage of their lives. This is especially true for those with cancer and for those in hospice and palliative care. Information can be returned to the person in a shortened version and shows that you have been listening attentively and also allows them to correct anything that has been misunderstood.

## Reflecting

Reflecting is where you focus on the feelings of the person. It allows the person to feel what they are indeed expressing, by hearing it come back from yourself. This can help them to identify any further feelings.

## Clarifying

During the first meeting with someone, it is often the case that there is a mixed and jumbled amount of information. Your role is to clarify with the person any information given is correct.

## Summarising

Summarising is where you give a brief outline of the main points. This is done at the end of the consultation and gives a complete picture of all the concerns, issues, and facts.

The difference between summarising and paraphrasing is that summarising deals with what has been said overall.

In going back to building rapport, it is very clear that in most communication situations, our postures, expressions, eye contact and tone of voice are of much more significant meaning than the words that we use.

To communicate effectively, it is of the most upmost importance to have the skill of rapport and understand the person correctly. This does not mean that you have to agree with them but shows that you are listening to them; they then feel that they have been understood.

Rapport can also be created by matching and mirroring someone else's body language and voice tone. This is called pacing, and from this, you can lead the person into the space you need for the best hypnotic trance-like state.

Here are some examples of matching and mirroring:

## Body

- Facial expressions
- Hand movements
- Eye movements
- Breathing

## Voice

- Volume
- Tone
- Pitch
- Tempo

## Personalising scripts

As human beings, we all appear to be very similar, but we are very different in a number of ways. We all have many likes and dislikes and come from many different cultural backgrounds, along with being brought up in different environments. This has led to our personal belief system and helps make us who we are. We are all very different and all unique in our own way.

In hypnosis, you will be communicating with language (verbal), and this is done with messages and suggestions, and in order to write the best possible script for the person that you are treating hypnosis with, you must work closely with them to understand their lives, their likes and dislikes, as well as their personality; this will ultimately lead you to gain their trust and to assist them in reaching a suitable state of hypnosis for the work to happen.

It is important to understand how our brains work to enable us to work in the best way. Read the following:

- Brains learn at great speed.
- Brains will externalise any instructions that has been given internally—which means the way people behave and react on the outside is a direct representation of their thinking internally. *You are what you think you are.*

- Brains leave and return to the present moment—which means that whatever the brain is taking in, it has the ability to retract from the present moment and do something else.
- Brains create our mental state—the body and mind are interlinked and inseparable.
- Brains do not stop—brains go backwards and forwards and around an issue; for example, if we cannot sleep because we are worried or excited, it is caught between a positive—and negative-thought process.
- Brains make sense of experience.
- Brains represent experiences from all our senses—this about 'modalities' being the first language of our minds (we will cover this in more detail in this part of the book).

The brain is divided into two main sections called hemispheres, which contain complementary abilities which are 'left brain' and 'right brain'. When and how you prefer to access the abilities of these hemispheres does determine your personality and behavioural patterns.

Logic and 'correctness' are of the left-brain hemisphere, and intuition and creativity are regarded as right-brain hemisphere skills. As a note of interest, because left-brain modes are more easily evaluated, schools do tend to favour left-brain modes of thinking; they then downplay the right-brain activities.

Left-brain people focus on logical thinking, analysis, and accuracy.

Right-brain people focus on feeling and creativity.

## Left-brain hemisphere

- Intellectual
- Objective
- Analyse
- Facts
- Deconstruct
- Detail focused
- Judgement
- Perfecting
- Yang (male energy)
- Language skills

## Right-brain hemisphere

- Intuitive
- Subjective
- Synthesise
- Concepts
- Connect the dots
- Bigger picture
- Perception
- Accepting
- Yin (female energy)
- Musical appreciation

## Modalities and representations

Our brain receives information from all our senses, and it represents it internally in a way that allows us to assess it and whether or not we need to act on these experiences or indeed store them for future reference. The senses which are referred to are sight, hearing, feeling, smelling, and tasting. All these senses are used, but we all have a favourite, which we are more comfortable with.

This all fits in to writing your hypnotherapy scripts, and if you can ascertain your patient's favourite modality, you can talk to them in the way that they will feel the most comfortable. When writing the induction (PMR or progressive muscle relaxation), it is beneficial to use all the senses, starting with the emphasis on their favourite modality and then introducing the others; this will create a safe and comfortable space for them, and by using the other modalities later on in the induction, it will be able to give the opportunity to enhance the experience and be able to expand boundaries and self-limiting beliefs.

Each of the modalities has representations in the person's physiology, language, behaviour, eye movement, and, even possibly, their preferences in leisure and work. A person will find one of the senses easier to imagine, and this, in turn, will create a comfort zone for them.

## Kinaesthetic (feeling)

This represents our own feeling system, both internally and externally. It can also include how we feel about something, namely, our own emotions. Kinaesthetic people will often tune into other people's emotions very quickly even before they speak to them. The kinaesthetic system is used when we feel an emotion, when we touch something, or when we are engaging in a physical activity. It is a fact that many of the people favouring this modality often enjoy sports and other 'feeling' activities.

Kinaesthetic people are those that touch everything before they buy something without thinking about their own actions.

## Kinaesthetic words

With this modality, the following words may be used from them and also in writing your scripts (there are many you can use, but I have only included some as a reference for you):

- Cool or cooling
- Touch or touching
- Move or moving
- Heavy, heavier, heaviest
- Hold or holding
- Smooth or smoothly

## Kinaesthetic phrases

- I know how you feel
- Hold on a moment
- Put your finger on it
- Pull some strings
- Smooth as silk

## Voice tone and breathing

Those in this modality may have a soft, lower, or deeper tone to their voice and speak with pauses in their speech. They may also breathe naturally deeper from their abdomens.

## Postures and gestures

Rounded shoulders, relaxed muscles, and their gestures are focussed to their mid or lower body.

## Visual (sight)

Visual thinking puts people in the realm of visual daydreams, fantasy, and imagination. We can all visualise, but those who do not have this as their primary modality will find it more difficult to do so. Visual people may be interested in drawing, designing, and TV (films, etc.).

## Visual language words

- Imagine
- Look or looking
- Watch or watching
- Colour or colouring
- Bright
- See or seeing

## Visual phrases

- I see what you mean
- Looks good to me
- Above and beyond
- Crystal clear
- Bird's-eye view
- Blown out of proportion

## Voice, tone, and breathing

Visual people do generally speak faster in a high but clear tone. Their breathing is often naturally shallower in the top part of the chest.

## Posture and gestures

Visual people may hold their body in a less-than-relaxed way and are often (although not always) thinner in their body type.

## Auditory (hearing)

This modality is associated with listening internally to sounds that include music and speech, as well as imagining other sounds. So, for example, if you were imagining a piece of music, you will be imagining it with your auditory system. These people will be on the phone and have music playing often (it would have to be of their own choosing). They will be upset and also unable to concentrate if the sounds are not to their own liking (they may be sensitive to obtrusive noise). They may be interested in languages, music, and lecturing.

## Auditory language words

- Discuss
- Harmony or harmonise
- Remark or remarking
- Say or saying
- Alarm or alarming
- Buzz or buzzing

## Auditory language phrases

- What did you say
- On the same wavelength
- Speak your mind
- Loud and clear
- Listen to yourself

## Vice tone and breathing

Auditory people will speak in a melodious style. Their breathing will be even and will focus on the centre of their chest.

## Posture and gesture

Auditory people are often of a medium body type and sometimes tilt their head to one side. They may also exhibit rhythmic body movements at times.

Both olfactory and gustatory are considered to be secondary modalities, but I have a strong opinion that they are just as much value, if not more so, than the other types of modalities. Taste and smell have a very profound effect on our emotions, and we can have a very good connection to it on an everyday level.

## Olfactory (smell)

### Olfactory words

- Nose
- Fragrance
- Rotten
- Mould or mouldy
- Sour or soured
- Stink or stinky

### Olfactory phrases

- I smell a rat
- A nose for business
- Sniffing things out
- Sweet smell of success
- That behaviour stinks

## Gustatory (taste)

**Gustatory words**

- Chew or chewing
- Sweet or sweetness
- Spice or spicy
- Sugar or sugary
- Thirst or thirsty

**Gustatory phrases**

- Bitter experience
- Stomach-turning
- Mouth-watering
- A taste for the good life
- Bitter disappointment

This is where people think mostly in language and symbols. People who are of this modality will often stand up tall and have their arms crossed.

There is one other modality and that is auditory digital (internal dialogue). Their breathing pattern is shallow and slightly restrictive, and speech is fairly monotone, and information is logical and straight to the point.

Using all the senses is the best way to achieve a deep hypnotic state, and, in using all the senses, it is called compounding.

## A word about lateral eye movements (LEM)

It is possible to identify a person's thinking process by their eye movements. We all tend to move our eyes according to which representation system (modality) we are accessing. In most cases, this is a very reliable indicator of how a person is thinking and is of great benefit in assessing and writing your scripts.

*In general, we tend to look upwards (to the left or the right) when we are using a visual thought process.*

*In general, we tend to look ahead (or side to side) when we are using a auditory thought process.*

*In general, we tend to look down for kinaesthetic thought process.*

The following is a typical pattern for a right-handed person as you look at them:

| | | | |
|---|---|---|---|
| Visual construct | | | Visual remembered |
| Auditory construct | *Eyes* | *Eyes* | Auditory remembered |
| Kinaesthetic | | | Internal dialogue |

A word of note is that construct is constructing an idea or thought, and remembered is remembering an idea or thought.

## Permissive and authoritarian style scripts

There are two recognised styles of hypnotic induction. They are permissive and authoritarian.

## Permissive

The permissive style is nurturing and provides an internal environment of safety, allowing for choice at all times. The words used are caring and always leave choice, for example, as follows:

- You may like to close your eyes
- You could make yourself as comfortable as possible

When employing the permissive style in writing your scripts, you give them a sense of safety and do not trap them or boss them around in any way. In this way, the scripts can often be more imaginative, using metaphors which incorporate varying amounts of imagination.

The permissive style of writing is most suited to clients who are caring, eager to please or very imaginative, and do not challenge ideas and realities.

## An example of a permissive-style PMR

'now . . . as you are in your very own special place . . . you are enjoying the experience of being there . . . taking in the whole picture in your mind . . . with all of your senses . . . you can easily see yourself in your very own special house . . . your very own special house . . . the house is just as you would like to imagine it . . . the house can be anywhere you wish . . . any size you wish . . . any shape you wish . . . any colour you wish . . . the house can be whatever you would like it to be . . .

In this house . . . you feel calm and safe . . . safe and calm . . . and as you drift deeper and deeper . . . deeper and deeper . . . you imagine that you are standing in your very own special house right now . . . you can look around you . . . where would you like to go . . . what can you see . . . you may like to see what the house is made of . . . what colour is it . . . what style is it . . . and as you do so . . . use all your senses . . . you can experience it . . . you can feel it . . . you can see it . . . you can hear it . . . you can smell it . . . the atmosphere . . . the décor . . . enjoy this house . . . this is your place . . . your very own special place . . .

You could . . . if you want to . . . allow yourself to go into the lounge . . . and everything there is perfect . . . all around you is just perfect . . . this is your dream home . . . this really is your very own special place . . .'

You can see from this script that it is permissive in style and the messages will be sent to the subconscious. The house is a symbol of the person themselves and any behaviour changes will be made in the house and then be brought back with them into their everyday life and consciousness.

## Authoritarian

When writing scripts in the authoritarian style they will be direct and logical with no choices. They will be to the point and not littered with metaphors. The images will be based on the person remaining in control and on the power of the mind.

Phrases used might be like :

- Use your powerful subconscious mind to imagine that you are relaxing in this chair
- Now close your eyes knowing that you will always be in control

This style can seem quite harsh but is very, very effective for the right person. Some people like to be told what to do and respond very well to the suggestions that are being made.

## An example of an Authoritarian style PMR

'Now . . . just close your eyes and move yourself into the most comfortable position you can . . . throughout this experience you will always be in control . . . you will always be aware . . . the natural state that you will achieve is completely OK for you . . . it will assist you to make the changes that you have come here today to achieve . . .

Now . . . start by concentrating on your breathing . . . my voice . . . all the outside noises will be irrelevant to you . . . you will use your powerful ability . . . of your mind to concentrate on your breathing . . . my voice will be helping you to achieve the state most beneficial for you . . . now you will relax your body . . . still concentrating on my voice . . . now you relax your body . . . from the muscles in the top of your head to the tips of your toes . . .

You know start at the top of your head . . . and relax now . . . always in control . . . you have an idea now of what you are doing . . . as you concentrate on your breathing . . . deepening your breathing . . . you now move down your body . . . always in control . . . and your powerful subconscious will allow your body to relax completely . . . now you are relaxed . . . your mind is ready to make those suggestions . . . that are put to you . . . to assist you in the healing process . . .'

You can see that it is direct and straight to the point, but always allows the person to remain in control.

## A word of caution

The above scripts are only a guideline for your use, and there is always an exception to the rule where people are concerned. It is therefore really important to keep an open mind on your treatment plan and be fully aware that what a person is showing on the outside may not be always be a reflection of what they are feeling on the inside.

It is therefore very important that during the initial consultation that you assess the person's external appearance, their behaviours and their personality in a non—judge-mental way. Some people may respond to you in a way that they think that you will respond to best, and they may be affected by nerves.

The best way to assess them is to listen attentively and look at the person while you are talking to them and then see what style you think will be best for them, and if the script is not quite right for them, do not be afraid to adjust it accordingly. Quite often the best scripts are those with a combination of both permissive and authoritarian in style.

## The construction of a script

There are generally four parts to the hypnotic script, all of which play a very important role in the success of hypnosis.

They are as follows:

- **By achieving a physical and mental relaxation**—this can be done by the PMR or other inductions that we will cover in more detail in this part of the book)
- **The deepener**—this is where you take the person to a special place and take him or her further into a state of deeper hypnosis
- **The therapeutic suggestions**—this where you introduce all the suggestion work for the benefit of the person and the healing process
- **Reorientation or bringing back**—this is where you bring the person back to full awakening consciousness

## The PMR or relaxation induction

The PMR is a simple yet very effective part of the induction process whereby you relax the person by the power of suggestions. This is done by relaxing each group of the muscles in the body in turn. There are many ways in which you can do this, and with the power of your own imagination, you can adjust them to suit yours and the other person's style. (I have included earlier on in the book a sample of a PMR that I have written that has proved very effective and suits my own style of delivery.)

When delivering your own PMR, it should be done in a manner that is comfortable to you and, at the same time, relaxing the other person. The more comfortable and relaxed you are, the more comfortable and relaxed the other person will be.

It is best to deliver the PMR at a much slower than normal speaking speed, and this in itself can be quite challenging! The pace and tone will also be of great importance, so practice, practice, practice and you will be able to deliver the best PMR that you can do.

When delivering your PMR, always remember to do the following:

- Slow down; you need to remember the other person is enjoying it, and if you rush, you can make them feel tense and nervous.
- If you do get lost or confused in the words you are saying, you can stop and take a deep breathe, gather your thoughts and carry on; the chances are the person will not know that you got lost and thought it was part of the therapy session.
- When meeting new clients, I always invite them to see their very own special place. This creates a view of choice, and they can generally imagine a scene that they have created themselves to good effect (as the therapy sessions continue, you can then introduce more suggestions).
- Do not worry about what people will experience. Some will see just colours or experience feelings and sounds—whatever people experience is right for them and some do find it easier than others.
- When doing the reorientation or bringing back, you must get louder and faster when you count down or up with the sound of your voice.
- If in part of the process you have said that 'all other sounds will slowly disappear', then you must make sure that you say that all noises will come back to the person during the bringing back.

Now I personally favour the PMR for a great way of introducing the person to hypnosis and getting him or her in the relaxed state to do suggestion work and healing. However, it is important for you to know that there are many other ways of doing the induction, and I will briefly explain a few of them (below is a list of just a few of them, and the list is by no means endless).

## Rapid inductions

Rapid inductions have a great part in long-term therapy, and they do not take up so much time as a PMR. However, it is important to get to know the person better before using this type of induction. There are many variations and styles, and it is essential that you use one that is best suited to your technique and style.

## Eye-focus induction

The eye-focus induction is a very effective method for people who find it difficult to relax or are sceptical about the process.

## The following is a rapid pain induction (eye-focus)

'Now . . . now I would like you to look at your right hand . . . and on the palm of your right hand, I would like you to imagine a small . . . tiny . . . coloured spot . . . in the middle of your hand . . . and as you focus on that spot in your hand . . . , your eyes follow that spot as you move your hand to one side, then the other . . . and as you focus more and more on that spot in your hand . . . , you feel your eyelids begin to close . . . You can feel the muscles relax around your eyes . . . and when you are ready . . . , your eyes begin to close all by themselves . . . They close and stay firmly shut . . . and as they close . . . you can now place your palm of your hand down . . . to somewhere that is more comfortable to you . . .

Your eyelids are so relaxed that even if you wanted to, you could not open them . . . and when you are quite sure that you cannot open them . . . , I invite you to try and open them . . . but the more you try . . . the harder the eyes stay firmly closed and shut . . . The wonderful feeling of total relaxation now spreads all over your face and head . . . down your neck and shoulders . . . down through your arms and into your hands and fingers . . . relaxing every muscle and tendon that it washes over . . .

Now that wonderful relaxing feeling is moving down your body through your chest and back . . . over your stomach and into your hips . . . thighs . . . knees . . . shins . . . calves and now into your feet all the way down to your toes . . .

Your body is so relaxed . . . so very relaxed . . . and now that your body is totally relaxed, you are going to relax your mind . . . and when I ask you to . . . I want you to say silently to yourself in your mind . . . say silently to yourself the following . . . one hundred . . . ninety-nine . . . ninety-eight . . . ninety-seven . . . ninety-six . . . and as you count down, the picture in your mind's eye begins to fade . . . to fade further and further away . . . It fades away so feint that you can't see . . . or remember . . . any more numbers . . .

Now . . . now you have told me earlier . . . that you have some pain . . . some discomfort in your stomach area . . . and I invite you to see a small dial . . . in your mind's eye . . . like one you would see on a cooker . . . with the numbers running down from nine to one . . .

At the moment, it is set on the number five . . . and as the numbers increase . . . so the discomfort increases . . .

Now I would like you to turn that dial back down to number five . . . now down to four . . . three . . . two . . . and you feel the discomfort dissolve until by one . . . it has all gone . . .

Can you feel that . . . the pain has gone . . . and you again repeat the same process . . . up . . . and now down . . . and you feel the discomfort just melt away . . . you can now do this at any time you like . . . and in the future, whenever you feel too much discomfort . . . you just imagine the dial on any part of your body that is causing concern and just turn it down . . .'

Bring safely back . . .

## Handshake-method induction

This method takes a lot of practice and a lot of confidence and is best practised very frequently. You will have to watch out for the eyes starting to blink or close as this is a signal to raise the arm a little higher to reinforce the feelings. Please bear in mind that the initial up-and-down movements should be about three inches up and down.

'Now I would like you to put your arm out to me as if we are about to shake hands . . . (you now take the person's hand as if you were going to shake their hand but keeping his or her hand straight) . . . and now I would like you to look at me for just a little while . . . and as you do so . . . , you focus on me and listen to my voice . . . and you listen to what it is I have to say . . . and as you look at me . . . allow things to happen . . . just allow things to happen naturally . . . (you now can raise the person's arm and lower it down by about three inches either way)

And as I raise and lower your arm . . . , you notice there is a little drowsiness . . . feeling . . .

Around your eyes . . . and each time I raise your arm upward . . . , that heavy feeling in your eyes gets stronger . . . and stronger . . . and as they close even more . . . , they begin to close shut . . . they begin to close down all the way . . .'

You can now use the script for suggestion work according to the person's needs.

## The anchor or trigger induction

This type of induction does have a role to play in hypnosis. It is of the upmost importance that you have a good knowledge of the person you are working with and is another way of installing a trance-like state very quickly. I have included the word 'anchor' in the style of induction because it symbolises an anchoring of the person's positive feelings and emotions which then enables him or her to feel safe and secure, which then proves very effective when combined with the 'trigger' word.

The 'trigger' itself can be anything that the person can focus on. It can simply be a touch on his or her head or hand or a click of the fingers. Some people do respond better to a word such as 'calm' or 'relax'.

The way you do this is to hypnotise them in the normal way, and during the 'suggestion stage' of hypnosis install the trigger in the following way:

'Now . . . now the next time you come to see me for hypnosis, I will say the words . . ."calm now" (or whatever the trigger word or action you will use) to you three times . . . one after the other in this way . . . and if it is safe for you to do so . . . and only if it is safe for you to do so . . . , you will easily find that when I say "calm now" (or whatever the trigger word or action you will use) the very first time . . . , you will find yourself immediately in a relaxed and calm state . . . just as you are calm and relaxed now . . . and when I say " calm now" (or whatever the trigger word or action you will use) for the second time, you will go even deeper . . . even deeper . . . into this wonderful state . . ."calm now" (or whatever the trigger word or action you will use) and when I say it for the next and following time . . . , you will go deeper and deeper into relaxation . . . more deeply relaxed than you have ever felt before . . ."calm now" (or whatever the trigger word or action will be you will use) . . .'

You can then bring the person out of hypnosis in the normal way. You will then be able to go on the next hypnosis session. Use the words 'When it is safe to do so . . . calm now' to put them into a trance-like state, feeling calm and relaxed, very quickly.

## Another popular method is to use the candle induction

'I would now like you to imagine a single candle which is lit . . . and now focus your mind on the flame of the candle. Notice the flickering and dancing of the flame as the yellows and reds swirl around . . .

Keep the candle in your mind as you go very gently . . . and very deeply . . . into a deep . . . deep . . . state of total relaxation . . . and as the flame flickers and dances . . . dances and flickers . . . , you may begin to notice a halo running around the flame . . . The more you focus on the candle . . . the more of the halo that you see . . .

And if . . . if you find that your mind begins to wander . . . , you can bring it back in . . . back to the focus of the candle . . . the flickering . . . flames . . . yellows . . . and reds . . . swirling around . . . the halo of the candle . . .

And now . . . now as you keep the flame of the candle there in your mind . . . , I will count down from ten to one . . . and as I do so . . . , each number will make you ten times more comfortable and relaxed than you are now . . .

Ready now . . .
Ten . . .
Nine . . .
Eight . . .
Seven . . .
Six . . .
Five . . .
Four . . .
Three . . .
Two . . .
One . . .
Deeply . . . deeply relaxed . . .
Zero . . .

You are now very deeply relaxed . . . and each and every suggestion that I make . . . will go deeply into your very powerful subconscious mind . . .'

## The deepener

The deepener is what you will use following the initial induction; this will deepen the trance-like state. There are many ways to do this, but the important thing to remember is to make sure the transition from the induction to the deepening stage flows as much as possible, without losing the trance-like state you have created.

Using the deepener will increase suggestibility and will enable you to use more imagination and imagery. The deepener is also very good for the person you are working with; it allows them to feel even more calm and relaxed, and the more calm and relaxed you can make them feel, the better the powerful subconscious will take on board any positive suggestions that you make.

You need to make sure that any imagery and the style of the deepener is most suited to the person you are working with. Some people may not appreciate any use of stairs, for example, if they have had a bad experience on a set of stairs at some point in time. Another example could be the use of lifts; some people may again have had a bad experience and may be frightened and scared of lifts.

The purpose of the deepener is to bypass the CCF (critical conscious faculty), which is done by relaxing the conscious mind, which allows for greater imagination to take place. Some people may even feel that they are floating or sinking, all in a good way though!

Deepeners can be used with or without imagery, but it is essential to keep using suggestions to allow deeper and deeper relaxation.

## Some examples of deepeners

### The candle

'Imagine in your mind's eye a single candle which is lit . . . Now focus your very own mind on the flame of that single candle . . . You notice the flickering . . . and dancing of the flame as the colours begin to swirl . . . swirl . . . around . . . You may notice reds . . . yellows . . . blues . . . purples . . . whites . . . or maybe even other colours . . . You see all the wonderful . . . beautiful . . . colours . . . swirling . . . dancing . . . around one another . . .

And now . . . now as you keep the candle in your very own mind . . . , you gently begin to relax deeper and deeper . . . deeper and deeper . . . deeply more relaxed as you watch the flames of that one single candle . . . swirling . . . dancing . . . around one another . . .

And as you keep the image of the candle in your mind . . . , I will count down from ten to one . . . and each number will allow you to relax ten times more . . . ten times more relaxed than you are right now . . .

Ten . . .
Nine . . .
Eight . . .
Seven . . .
Six . . .
Five . . .
Four . . .
Three . . .
Two . . .
One . . .
Deeply . . . deeply relaxed . . .
Zero . . .

Now . . . now notice the wax of the candle . . . as you see the trickle of melting wax . . . begin to move down . . . down . . . down the candle . . . and as it does so . . . , you can become aware of the melting sensations within your own peaceful body . . . and as you begin to relax more and more . . . , you can see the melting wax . . . as it touches the candle holder . . . and as it merges with the base of the candle holder . . . , you become deeper . . . deeper . . . deeper relaxed . . .

You are now very deeply relaxed . . . and with each and every suggestion that I make . . . , it will go deeply . . . deeply into your mind . . . and as it does so . . . , you will feel safe and comfortable . . . comfortable and safe . . . and with every word that I say . . . , you will become deeply . . . deeply relaxed . . .'

## The star

'As you become more and more relaxed . . . , you may find that your mind wanders away to some pleasant thoughts . . . and that is fine . . . That is perfectly fine . . . and because your very own inner mind continues to listen . . . and enjoy the growing sense of peace . . . harmony . . . and tranquillity that is growing and developing within you right now . . .

And because you know those wonderful feelings that you have when you are sleeping soundly . . . and how you wish that you could just be left to doze and rest . . . , you can remember how you felt when you laid lazily on a lawn . . . or a beach in the sun . . . perhaps . . . even drifting in and out of a dozing sleep . . . yawning . . . and just wanting to stay where you were . . .

And in a moment, I am going to count slowly back . . . slowly back from ten to zero . . . and as I do so . . . , you will find that you will relax more and more . . . with each number that I count . . . until you feel as you did on those lazy occasions in the past . . . and just as deeply relaxed . . . deeply relaxed as you were then . . .

Ready now . . .
Ten . . . you feel yourself going down . . .
Nine . . . lazily drifting down . . .
Eight . . . relaxing more and more . . .
Seven . . . going deeper down . . .
Six . . . deeper and deeper . . . deeper and deeper . . .
Five . . . halfway to relaxation . . .
Four . . . and that wonderful . . . comfortable feeling . . .
Three . . .
Two . . . almost there now . . .
One . . .
Zero . . .

And now . . . now I want you to imagine that you are looking up into a beautiful night sky . . . and that you can see . . . in the distance . . . a star . . . you can see one beautiful . . . solitary . . . silvery star . . . shining down . . . out of a velvety black night sky . . . and that one star . . . is millions and millions of miles away . . .

And as you focus your gaze entirely on that one . . . solitary . . . silver star . . . , you begin to notice that it begins to twinkle . . . and as it twinkles . . . , you become more and more relaxed . . . more peaceful . . . more calm . . .

And as you continue to listen to the sound of my voice . . . , you feel yourself becoming sleepier and sleepier . . . sleepier and sleepier . . . You begin to drift deeper and deeper . . . and you may almost feel like you are dropping off to sleep . . . because you are so relaxed . . . so relaxed . . . so relaxed . . .'

## The lift

'I would now like you to imagine that you are entering a lovely large lift . . . The doors open and you step inside . . . and the lift is large and roomy . . . and very . . . very comfortable . . . On one side of the walls, you notice a panel . . . and on this panel, there are buttons . . . all marked from ten to g . . . and g represents the ground floor . . . while all the numbers above it . . . represent all the other floors . . .

Once you are inside the lift . . . , the doors close gently behind you . . . and you then press a button . . . and as you reach each floor . . . , the button will light up . . . You begin to descend . . . and you feel yourself going down . . . going down . . .

The ninth-floor button lights up . . . and the doors do not open . . . They remain closed as you continue to drop deeper down . . . deeper down to the eight floor . . . and as you reach the eight floor . . . , again the doors remain closed . . . and you feel very comfortable and relaxed here . . . and now . . . now the lift goes further and further down . . . down to the seventh floor . . .

Pause . . .

Deeper and deeper . . . deeper and deeper . . . down to the sixth floor . . .

Pause . . .

Even deeper . . . even more deeper . . . as you reach the fifth floor . . . becoming even more aware of how comfortable and relaxed you now are . . .

Going down . . . going down to the fourth floor . . . and once again the button lights up . . . and the door remains closed . . .

Further down you go now... further down to the third floor... going deeper... really going deeper inside yourself...

Second floor... and now the first...

And as you reach the first floor, the doors open... but you remain inside... because you are aware that there is an even deeper level of relaxation... a relaxation that is known as 'the basement of relaxation'... and the lift now begins to sink deep... deep... deep down... relaxing more and more... more and more...

You now go past the ground floor... and deeper down... deeper down to 'the basement of relaxation... And as the lift touches the ground..., it comes to a gentle... halt and stops... The doors open... and you step outside... into your very own special place...'

## Best friend method

This deepener is a variation of Milton Erickson's 'My Friend John' method. This deepener works very well for resistant people, as most people like to help others or show them what to do; consequently the person, in showing his best friend how to go into a trance, goes into trance himself or herself.

This is what to say...

'See that chair over there? I would like you to imagine that your best friend is sitting there, waiting to be hypnotised, and that you are the one who is going to show them how to do it. So now form an awareness of how your friend looks, whilst sitting there. Give the instructions to your friend after me (in your mind, if you wish).

Tell your best friend to close his eyes. Tell him to relax the tiny muscles around the eyes. Are they relaxed? Good. Now tell him to relax all the facial muscles and very slowly, very gradually, talk him through relaxing the rest of his body, working down from the head to the toes and the shoulders to the fingertips.'

Give a long pause to allow the person to carry out this instruction, intercepted with 'that's right' 'good', 'relax', very softly. Watch the person for muscle relaxation and change of skin colour. Then continue with the suggestion change of the script.

## The staircase

'As you become more and more relaxed . . . , you are aware of a beautiful staircase . . . an ornate staircase . . . polished all the way down . . . running down to a deep . . . rich . . . beautiful . . . rich carpet . . . underneath your bare feet . . . and as you look down the staircase . . . , you notice that there are ten steps leading down . . . ten steps leading down to your very own special place . . .

And in your very own special place . . . , these steps will lead you down into a deep relaxation . . . a deep . . . deep relaxation . . . and in a moment, I would like you to walk down those steps with me . . . and as we do so . . . , I will count them off one at a time . . . and the deeper down you go . . . , the more comfortable and relaxed you will become . . .

And when you are ready to walk down those stairs . . . , I would like you to gently place your hand on the banister . . . and begin to slowly descend those set of stairs . . . as I slowly count them off from ten to one . . . Ready now . . .

Ten . . . deeply relaxed . . . deeply . . . comfortably relaxed . . .
Nine . . . even more deeply . . . deeply relaxed . . .
Eight . . . even more and more comfortably . . . deeply relaxed . . .
Seven . . . deeply relaxed . . . deeply comfortably relaxed . . .
Six . . . even more relaxed . . .
Five . . . more and more relaxed . . .
Four . . . deeply relaxed . . . deeply comfortably relaxed . . .
Three . . . more and more relaxed . . . more and more relaxed . . .
Two . . . almost to the bottom now . . .

One . . . going deeper and deeper . . . deeper and deeper . . . all the way down to a deeper . . . comfortable place . . .

You are now standing at the bottom of the set of stairs . . .'

## Therapeutic suggestions

The suggestion phase is next, and this is where the suggestion work is introduced. The best place to do this is in the person's very own special place. It is important that the special place is somewhere where the person will not be disturbed and must produce a positive feeling for them. It is in this special place that they will have an increased receptivity to further suggestions. Once a peaceful feeling is established, it will be possible for the person to be responsive to imagery, which will reinforce and support posthypnotic suggestions.

There are some guidelines when you write your own suggestions. They are as follows:

- Always keep direct suggestions simple and concise.
- You can repeat suggestions.
- Use words that are positive, rather than negative.
- If you are using guided imagery suggestions, you must make sure that if you are using a location or special place from the past, you do not associate any slightest negative feelings with it.
- The more intensely you can suggest an image or scene, the more successful the suggestion will be.
- The most important parts of the scene should be associated with peacefulness.
- The voice that you use in your hypnotic script is of the upmost importance. The voice alone can produce a trance-like state and is extremely important to the entire hypnotic experience. The voice can be forceful and commanding, or it can be soothing and melodic, but the tone and volume will play a big part as well.
- Words are sometimes distorted to achieve a special and desired effect. For example, 'Feel those muscles loooooose and relaxed, feel those calf muscles loooooose and relaxed'. These types of word distortion are beneficial when someone is having a difficult time relaxing and getting comfortable.
- The whole level of the voice changes when you use a raised pitch. This pitch will enable you to penetrate the relaxed state of mind. This pitch will allow for an emphasis to be placed on suggestions such as 'And now you will feel no pain in your left leg'.
- When you use silent pauses, it allows time for a response to a suggestion, for example, 'Now take a deep breath . . . now exhale . . .' It is essential when using the pause that you allow enough time for each response to happen.
- Metaphors are a great way of using suggestions in the script. If you can tell the person a story and make it believable, then they can take the suggestions on board more easily. It is a very powerful way of using suggestions if used properly.

## Reorientation and bringing back

When bringing someone back from the trance-like state, it is important to bring a feeling of well-being back for the person. This should be done gently and not in an abrupt way, which may cause drowsiness or a headache.

This can be done either by using the counting-up or counting-down method.

For example, 'Enjoy your special place for a short while and then I will count from one to ten . . . and as I do so, you can begin coming back to full consciousness . . . coming back feeling refreshed as if you had a long rest . . . Begin to come back now . . . one . . . two . . . coming up . . . three . . . four . . . five . . . six . . . seven . . . eight . . . nine . . . and now ten . . . You can open your eyes and come all the way back . . . feeling great . . . feeling calm and relaxed . . .'

## Fears and Phobias

When treating people with cancer and those in hospice and palliative care, one of the stumbling blocks they might find in their treatment is fear or phobia. The physical reaction to this could be one of mild to intense. This could include the symptoms such as sweaty palms, erratic heartbeat, nausea, increased muscle tension, shortness of breath, blurred vision, and even fainting.

Fears and phobias could include the fear of needles and a fear of being sick with any treatment plan for example. In the treatment of such cases, it is very important to relax the person as much as possible before treating the condition.

You must be able to take the fear or phobia seriously, as for the person who is suffering from this condition, the fear or phobia is very real.

In general, the majority of phobias are generated from one of the five following causes:

- **The phobia may be the product of severe stress**

Stress may have been repressed for a long time or to such a degree that it surfaces in another form, that of an irrational fear.

- **The phobia may be the product of a series of experiences occurring over a period of years, which would have built up into an anxiety state**

This may be because of an accumulation of distressing events which cause a sense of dread and fear. This also may include a series of negative experiences that reinforce each other, which results in a phobia that can transfer to other areas of life.

- **Your phobia may be the product of a fear of fear**

If you have a fear of panic and fear itself, it is a very real phobia. By anticipating panic, you will raise your stress levels and the fear of fear can turn into a destructive cycle.

- **Your fear or phobia may have been transferred to you from somebody else**

This can come from someone with whom you are in close contact—a friend, a neighbour, or a stranger. If you notice they have a fear of needles, for example, you may then also begin to have that fear yourself.

- **Your fear or phobia may be because of your past experience**

A painful emotional experience from the past can produce a fear of that same situation. This trauma can be either conscious or subconscious, meaning that you may be aware of the original cause of the fear or it may have been buried and you have no conscious memory of it.

## Ways to deal with phobias when writing your script

- **You could identify the relevant event that caused the fear and then cut any emotional ties to it**

This technique is called 'regression' and is really best done by an experienced hypnotherapist and is not suitable for everybody. If the fear came from an extremely traumatic situation, it may bring up other emotional problems to the surface. It is, however, a very powerful technique, and I strongly urge you to seek out a qualified hypnotherapist if this option is intended to be used.

- **You could confront your fear when experiencing it as a non-threatening experience**

This is a very good way of dealing with a fear or phobia; you can see yourself re-enacting the experience from a safe vantage point, where no harm will come to you. You could use the words such as the following:

'I would like you know to imagine . . . imagine that you are face-to-face with your fear . . . No harm will come to you . . . You feel calm and relaxed . . . relaxed and calm . . . You feel at ease with yourself . . . You feel at ease with yourself . . . You are now smiling to yourself . . . You are smiling because your fear . . . your fear has lost all its strength . . . its importance . . . and from now on . . . from now on, you no longer need that fear . . . and you no longer want that fear . . . The fear is not real . . . You are no longer afraid of needles . . . and you are happy . . . you are very happy to allow the needle to be used . . . to be used for your own well-being and care . . . for your own highest good . . . your very own highest good.'

- **You could increase your self-confidence**

When working with fear or 'false evidence appearing real' as it is sometimes known as, fear is about something that may have or may have not happened in the past. It is something that has not happened in the present moment and, therefore, is not a real experience in the here and now. However, to some people, the fear is almost like it is happening to them at any given moment and appears to be 'very real'. A very good way of treating someone would be to work with his or her confidence.

You could, for example, use the following words:

'And now . . . now you are confident . . . you are very confident . . . You can face anything . . . you can really face anything . . . for now . . . now . . . this very moment in time . . . you have tremendous strength . . . tremendous strength and courage . . . and from now on . . . from now on from this moment in time . . . whenever you feel anxious and fear . . . you have . . . you have deep inside . . . within you . . . all the strength . . . and courage . . . that you need . . . you have all the strength and courage within you . . . All you have to do is ask . . . all you have to do is ask your higher self . . . to lovingly guide and protect you . . . to lovingly guide and protect you . . .'

**I have included some scripts for you to use which you may find useful when treating those with a fear or phobia**

# Fear of needles script

'And now as you relax deeper and deeper . . . deeper and deeper . . . in your very own special place . . . , I would like you to remember . . . to remember that in the past, you were worried . . . you were worried about needles . . . and the injection on the skin . . . In fact . . . the very thought of having an injection . . . would make your knees tremble like jelly . . . and all you wanted to do was run away . . . run away from the very situation that you were in . . .

Do you know . . . do you know that most people who are not afraid of needles . . . only find it mildly uncomfortable . . . and when they have the injection . . . they are calm and relaxed . . . relaxed and calm . . . ?

And do you know . . . do you know that the discomfort is so minimal . . . it is so minimal because of all the preparations . . . all of those preparations that those lovely nurses and doctors do . . . they can numb the nerves before they use the needle . . . so that you will only have a very mild discomfort . . . a very mild discomfort . . . ?

All you need to deal with . . . is to deal with the fear . . . the fear that you have . . . the fear that you have from a past experience . . . a past experience that you have found unpleasant . . . and because . . . and because you have learnt fear . . . , you can unlearn fear . . . and learn not to be fearful . . .

You have a wonderful imagination . . . and you can use that wonderful imagination to overcome that fear . . . You can be un-fearful of needles . . . un-fearful of injections . . . All you have to do . . . all you have to do is use that wonderful imagination of yours . . .

So now . . . now I would like you to imagine . . . to imagine you are looking at a TV set in front of you . . . and on that TV set is a scene, a scene where you were having an injection . . . when you were having a needle being used for an injection . . .

And on this scene . . . you were calm and relaxed . . . relaxed and calm . . . and because you were calm and relaxed . . . relaxed and calm . . . , you had no fear . . . you had no fear of this injection . . . of this needle being inserted in your arm . . . You felt so calm and relaxed . . . relaxed and calm . . .

I would like you to watch this scene . . . watch this scene in front of you . . . You watch as you were no longer afraid . . . no longer afraid of the injection . . . no longer afraid of having the needle inserted into your arm . . .

And as you watch this scene . . . you watch this scene with the needle being inserted into your arm . . . calm and relaxed . . . relaxed and calm . . . no longer afraid . . . no longer afraid of that needle being inserted into your arm . . . and as this scene comes to an end . . . comes to an end . . . , I would like you to rewind this scene . . . rewind this scene . . . to the very beginning . . . the very beginning when you were sitting in that chair . . . waiting for your injection . . . waiting for that needle to go into your arm . . . You feel calm and relaxed . . . relaxed and calm . . .

And because you are calm and relaxed . . . relaxed and calm . . . you have no negative feelings . . . You have no negative feelings associated with needles . . . with having an injection into your arm . . . so now . . . now I would like you to play this scene again . . . to play this scene from the very beginning . . . to see yourself calm and relaxed . . . relaxed and calm . . . You have no fear . . . You have no fear associated with needles . . . You have no fear associated with having an injection in your arm . . .

And as you watch calm and relaxed . . . relaxed and calm . . . , I would like you to remember . . . to remember that feeling of being in your very own special place . . . that feeling of love . . . of joy . . . of happiness . . . and of peace . . . This really is your very own special place . . . your very own special place . . .

And because you are in your very own special place . . . , there is nothing . . . or nobody that can disturb your feeling . . . your feeling of being calm and relaxed . . . relaxed and calm . . . You are in control . . . You are in control of your feelings . . . You are in control of your very own feelings . . .

So now . . . now I would like you to play the scene once again . . . to play the scene in front of you . . . without any fear . . . without any fear of needles . . . without any fear of having an injection in your arm . . .

And as you watch this scene play in front of you . . . , you can see yourself . . . you can see yourself . . . without any fear . . . you are calm and relaxed . . . relaxed and calm . . . You have no fear of the needle . . . of the injection going into your arm . . .

And now . . . now I would like you to watch as you see the needle . . . You see the injection going into your arm . . . You have no fear . . . You have no fear . . . because you are calm and relaxed . . . relaxed and calm . . . and you watch as the needle is being taken out of your arm . . . You watch as you feel calm and relaxed . . . relaxed and calm . . .

You watch this scene in front of you come to an end . . . you watch as you see yourself no longer afraid . . . no longer afraid of an injection . . . of having a needle inserted into your arm . . . you watch as you are calm and relaxed . . . relaxed and calm . . .

And now . . . now from now on . . . whenever you have an injection . . . a needle in your arm . . . , you have no fear . . . You have no fear . . . and because you can say to yourself . . . you can say to yourself in that chair . . . I am calm and relaxed . . . relaxed and calm . . . You will not have any fear . . . any fear of having an injection . . . of having a needle in your arm . . .

So the very next time . . . the very next time you are sitting in that chair . . . , all you have to do is say to yourself . . . I am calm and relaxed . . . relaxed and calm . . . and everything will be fine . . . everything will just be fine . . .'

## Fear of doctors or operations (this is a regression script)

'And as you drift deeper and deeper . . . deeper and deeper . . . , you feel those wonderful feelings of peace and well-being . . . those wonderful feelings of calm . . . calm . . . calm . . .

It is as though nothing else matters right now . . . except for you and this beautiful feeling of relaxation . . . enveloping you like a cocoon of warmth . . . safety . . . and peace . . . and as you go deeper into this lovely . . . warm feeling . . . , you are just beginning to realise . . . You are just beginning to realise how . . . in the past . . . You worried unnecessarily . . . about seeing a doctor . . . or having an operation . . .

And I wonder . . . I wonder when you are going to change . . . when you are going to change your mind . . . to change and appreciate all the good work doctors . . . nurses . . .

Medical staff . . . do . . . They are your friends . . . They really are your friends . . . They are here to help you . . . and to help the people that you love . . .

There may have been many reasons . . . many good reasons to you . . . why . . . in the past you developed your fears . . . of doctors and the operations that they perform . . . that they perform so very well . . .

And because . . . because you are here . . . you are here in the safety of hypnosis . . . , I wonder if you would like to explore those fears now . . . now in the safety of hypnosis . . .

That's good . . . that's very good . . . , so now . . . now let us drift your mind back . . . drift your mind gently back . . . as though you are travelling through a tunnel . . . and as you go further back in time . . . past the more recent memories . . . , you are going further into gentle hypnotic rest . . . You are becoming younger and younger . . . smaller and smaller . . . drifting back through time . . . as though time does not exist . . . in the sense that we know of now . . .

And when you are there . . . when you are really there . . . back at that point in your life when your fear began . . . , I would like you to ask your subconscious mind . . . to ask . . . Was this the very first time that I felt that fear? . . . And if that was . . . , I would now like you to project that image . . . to project that memory on to an imaginary screen . . .

And as you watch . . . as you watch all those events of that moment in time . . . before your own eyes . . . from the very beginning . . . to the very end . . . , I want you to know . . . to know that you are perfectly safe . . . perfectly safe . . . here . . . right now . . . in this state of deep hypnosis . . . this very moment in time . . .

And because you are safe . . . and you can see from a comfortable distance . . . , you allow the scene to unfold before you . . . It is like watching a film . . . and you have full control . . . You can stop and examine any parts of that film . . . any experience that you wish . . . you have the controls in front of you . . . and you can . . . , if you so wish, stop the film any time that you so wish . . .

And when . . . when you have been through the scene once . . . , I would like you to repeat the exercise once again . . . and as you watch this film in front of you unfold . . . , you begin to notice . . . you begin to notice how the second time . . . you view this scene . . . it loses its intensity . . . You begin to feel more removed from those original feelings . . . Can you notice that? . . . Good . . . very good . . .

Now . . . now once again I would like you to play that scene again . . . and as you play that film . . . in front of you . . . before your very own eyes . . . , you notice how detached from that experience you are . . . how detached from that experience you are . . . right now . . . right now . . . this moment in time . . . You allow those feelings to float away . . . to float away . . . and as you watch . . . you watch as it fades with colour . . . losing its brightness . . . becoming dimmer and dimmer . . . dimmer and dimmer . . . fainter and fainter . . . fainter and fainter . . . as it slowly . . . gently . . . disappears . . . in front of your very own eyes . . .

And as that film . . . that scene fades away . . . so do your fears . . . your fears just dissolve . . . right now . . . in front of your very own eyes . . . and you no longer need those fears . . . Your fears about that event have now gone . . .

Now . . . now I would like you to create a new screen in your mind . . . and as you do so . . . , I would like you to project yourself on to this screen . . . just as though you were speaking to your doctor . . . just as though you were going for an operation . . . and as you do so . . . , you notice how calm and relaxed . . . relaxed and calm . . . you are . . . You watch . . . you watch as you see yourself sitting or lying . . . with your doctor beside you . . .

And you know . . . you know that this doctor is just an ordinary person . . . A friendly person . . . someone who wishes you no harm . . . a person who is your friend . . . someone who is trained to help you with any problems . . . any problems . . . that you may have . . .

The doctor in front of you . . . is just like any other normal human being . . . with all the same bodily functions as you . . . and even doctors have to visit another doctor . . . from time to time . . . with no fear . . . with no fear or worries . . .

And do you know . . . do you know that we all have a good side and a bad side from time to time . . . ? And if . . . in the past . . . you had any negative experience with a doctor . . . or a surgeon . . . or anybody else in the medical profession . . . , you know . . . deep in your very own heart . . . that is all it was . . . a negative experience with one person . . . and it certainly does not mean that everyone else will treat you in the same way . . .

So now . . . now let go of your old fear . . . or worry . . . or concern . . . for you now realise that it no longer serves any purpose in your life . . . any more . . . You know that we all deserve to be treated with respect . . . not just doctors . . .

but everyone they themselves treat . . . as a patient that you are . . . as a patient that you are . . .

And do you know . . . do you know that the doctors . . . the surgeons . . . can advise you . . . can advise you on the best treatment plan for you . . . ? They can treat you . . . in the best possible way . . . in the best possible way with your consent . . . , so do not be afraid . . . Please do not be afraid . . . for they really do have your best interests at heart . . .

And as you listen to the sound of my voice . . . more and more . . . more and more . . . , your very own subconscious is acting . . . and accepting . . . all those suggestions that you have received . . . and that from now on . . . from this very moment in time . . . you are not afraid . . . or fearful . . . of receiving treatment from the doctor . . . surgeon . . . or anybody else . . . in the medical profession . . . You will find yourself becoming so much more confident . . . in every way . . . whenever you meet your doctor . . . or surgeon . . . They really do have your best interests at heart . . . They are the best people to help you . . . in your treatment plan ahead . . .

You feel happier and relaxed . . . and you will be happier and relaxed whenever it is time to see your doctor . . . your surgeon . . . in the coming times ahead . . . and the suggestions that I make . . . will grow stronger and stronger . . . with each and every passing day . . .'

## Fear of blood script

'And as you drift . . . further and further . . . further and further . . . , you drift into the deepest state of relaxation possible . . . and as you do so . . . , your very own subconscious mind is open . . . and receptive to the suggestions that you are about to hear . . . and even though . . . you may find your mind wandering from time to time . . . , you will hear everything that is said to you . . . at a deeper level of mind . . .

And today . . . today you are listening to me because you would like to overcome a fear of blood . . . and because you are here today . . . and because you want to overcome that fear . . . , you are already halfway there . . . The next half will be easy to you . . . as I guide you the rest of the way . . . to overcome your fear of blood . . .

Do you know . . . do you know that those people who suffer from fears and phobias . . . have proved themselves to be excellent hypnotic people . . . because they have . . . at some point in their lives . . . been negatively hypnotised in order to develop their fear . . . ?

So now . . . now we are going to visit your past . . . to learn why that fear established itself in you . . . so allow your mind to wander . . . to wander back in time . . . to feel a sense of yourself . . . getting younger and younger . . . younger and younger . . . going further and further . . . further and back in time . . . smaller and smaller . . . smaller and smaller . . .

And as you go back in time . . . , I wonder if you can recall the very first experience . . . that you remember . . . where you were afraid . . . or even cautious about seeing . . . or hearing about blood . . .

And as you continue to recall that experience . . . , I am going to count the numbers down from ten to one . . . and with each and every descending number . . . you will find yourself going further and further back in time . . .

Ready now . . . ?

Ten . . . going further back . . .

Nine . . . becoming younger and smaller . . .

Eight . . . you are deeply relaxed . . . going back . . . going back . . .

Seven . . . going back even further now . . .

Six . . . back you go . . . further and further back . . .

Five . . . and as you go back . . . if you begin to experience any discomfort . . . this means that you are getting closer and closer . . . closer and closer to the cause of that fear . . .

Four . . . further back you go . . . further and further back you go . . .

Three . . . you are now nearing that event . . .

Two . . . almost there . . .

One . . . just allow yourself to be totally relaxed . . . completely relaxed . . . You feel safe and calm . . . calm and safe . . .

And you realise . . . you realise that something happened to you . . . or even somebody else at this time that instilled a fear of blood within you . . . and because you feel calm and safe . . . safe and calm . . . , I would like you to allow your mind to absorb any sensations . . . experiences . . . thoughts . . . or anything else that connects itself to your fear of blood . . .

Slight pause . . .

Now . . . now I would like you to project everything that you can remember with this experience on to a large . . . white . . . flat screen . . . Notice all the bright colours . . . You begin to enhance any smells . . . any feelings . . . so that they are large and bright . . . and as you are resting here . . . looking at this screen in front of you . . . , you recall the events that caused you to fear blood . . .

And you know . . . you know what a totally irrational fear this is . . . for without blood . . . without blood, not one single person could even live . . . for blood is our very own life force . . . It is something that is to be respected and looked after . . . It is not something to be feared of . . .

And as you begin to realise this . . . , you notice how the screen is all tied up together by ropes and string . . . and in your hand is a pair of scissors . . . to cut right through those ropes and strings . . . and as you cut through those ropes and strings . . . , you notice immediately . . . straight away . . . that you feel free . . . and as you begin to feel more and more free of that fear . . . , you watch as the screen in front of you begins to fade away . . . into the distance . . . Your fear fades way into the distance . . .

And now you are free from that old fear of blood . . . From now on, you respect blood . . . Whether it is yours or somebody else's . . . you know now that your fear was based on a distorted memory . . . The initials of the word *fear* stand for *false evidence appearing real* . . . And that is all that they were . . . false evidence that created a needles fear . . .

Now . . . now I would like you to project yourself into the future . . . just a little bit into the future . . . and imagine yourself as being a blood donor . . . and feeling really proud of yourself . . . for donating your very own blood . . . knowing that it could save someone else's life . . . and you also know that you have overcome your fear . . . your fear of blood once and for all . . .

And now . . . now as each and every day passes . . . , you feel more and more comfortable . . . each and every time you think about blood . . . and this feeling creates within you . . . an amazing confidence . . . of yourself . . . you have conquered once and for all . . . your fear of blood . . . and you realise . . . you realise that you . . . and only you are responsible . . . that you are in control . . . and all these suggestions are firmly . . . deeply . . . embedded into your subconscious mind . . . stronger and stronger . . . with each and every passing day . . .'

## Fear of anaesthesia script

'And now . . . now in this very pleasant state of hypnosis . . . , your very own subconscious mind is open . . . is open and receptive to a new way of thinking and feeling . . . and because you have an upcoming operation . . . which involves anaesthesia . . . and surgery . . . , you have been having unwanted thoughts . . . about the procedure of surgery . . .

I want you to know . . . that the first thing I would like you to say . . . is to reassure you . . . that there are many millions of people who do undergo surgery . . . without any problems at all . . . and in only a very small amount of cases, there are any problems . . . which are . . . perhaps with the anaesthesia . . . and these cases are brought to light and examined . . . and this makes them appear to be a common experience . . . when, in fact, . . . in fact, they are quite rare . . .

And do you know . . . do you know that surgeons and anaesthetists must undergo years and years of training before they are allowed to practice in their chosen field of medicine . . . ? They know . . . and have been highly trained to know exactly what to do . . . and are very highly specialised in their area . . . and should they ever make a mistake . . . , they will most likely lose their livelihood . . . , so they must . . . and do . . . take extra special care for their very own well-being . . . just as they do with your very own well-being . . .

Allow your mind to go back . . . to go back to the many generations that came before you . . . who had to undergo surgery . . . without any anaesthetic . . . And I want you to realise . . . to realise how fortunate we are to be living in this day and age . . . where we have learned so much . . . and that modern medicine and technology is within reach to all of us . . . which was not the case all those years ago . . . Patients in those days . . . had to undergo surgery with no analgesia at all . . . or face an uncertain death . . .

There was, however, . . . in those days gone by . . . an alternative to anesthetic . . . although then it was not that well known . . . It was called hypnotherapy . . . and by using the power of hypnosis, you can do absolutely anything that you desire . . . including mimicking the effects of anesthetic . . . You could literally send it to a far-off place . . . away . . . away . . . away . . .

And this . . . this is what you are going to do during your operation . . . alongside . . . and with the normal anesthetic procedure . . . to make sure . . . to make sure that your surgery runs smoothly . . . and if . . . if . . . when it comes to the day of your operation . . . you are concerned . . . concerned in any way at all . . . over the effectiveness of your anesthetic . . . , then I would like you to talk to your consultant before the operation . . . so you can explain your feelings . . . and they will be able to check that all is well . . . and relax your mind . . . well before the operation procedure is to be carried out . . .

So now . . . now I would like you to cast your mind forward . . . forward to the day of your operation . . . You are lying on the bed . . . all dressed in a hospital gown . . . and medical staff . . . are all around you . . . getting yourself ready for surgery . . . and as the time approaches . . . , you feel calm and relaxed . . . relaxed and calm . . . and before the anaesthesia is even injected into you . . . , you send yourself . . . into a state of deep hypnosis . . . just like you are doing right now . . . right now into a state of deep hypnosis . . . You have a warm . . . comfortable feeling within you . . . and you are completely unaware of the things that are going on around you . . .

And when you have decided on your place to go . . . , you can go anywhere . . . anywhere in your mind . . . You can visit this place anytime you wish . . . It may be a tropical island . . . with palm trees and gentle waves splashing lazily up to the shoreline . . . It may be an old country house and garden . . . with honeysuckle and beautiful butterflies dancing in the air . . .

It doesn't matter which place that you choose . . . in your mind . . . as long as it is a place that is special to you . . . and you will stay in this place until after your operation . . . and after the effects of the anaesthesia has worn off . . . and because this is your very own special place . . . , you want to spend every moment that you can . . . here . . . in this very special place . . .

And when you are ready . . . when you are ready to wake up . . . and walk back up that staircase . . . back to reality . . . , you will be pleasantly surprised to hear how well the operation went . . . You hear the surgeon telling you . . . telling you that this was one of the best results he has done . . . He is really pleased with his work . . . and you feel so much better . . . You are pleased with yourself for comfortably . . . and confidently going through with this operation . . . It went smoothly and pain free . . . and these thoughts of calm and peace . . . run through your entire body . . . They are going to remain with you . . . They are going to remain with you . . . long after you wake up . . .'

## Visualisations

Using visualisations are a very good way of relaxing a person who needs to relax more and is feeling slightly nervous or tense. They are a great way of developing a script for the right person, and because they are used as a metaphor, they can really allow the person who is a bit resistant to hypnosis relax more and more. Everyone likes a good story and allowing their imagination to run away with them. A very deep trance-like state can be produced with the right script and read in the right way.

## Visualisation: Dolphin Dreamtime

'Imagine that you are standing at the entrance of a very deep cave . . . looking down . . . You can see the entrance of the cave . . . and it feels warm and inviting . . . inviting and safe . . .

There are many steps leading down . . . down into the cave . . . and you begin to walk down the steps . . . counting with me in your mind as we go down . . .

Thirty . . . twenty-nine . . . twenty-eight . . . twenty-seven . . . twenty-six . . . twenty-five . . . twenty-four . . . twenty-three . . . twenty-two . . . twenty-one . . . Twenty . . . You arrive at a small landing . . . and you walk across the landing . . . towards the next flight of steps . . . Nineteen . . . eighteen . . . seventeen . . . sixteen . . . fifteen . . . fourteen . . . thirteen . . . twelve . . . eleven . . . ten . . . and as you come to the next landing . . . , you begin to walk over to the final flight of steps . . . still counting with me . . . as we continue to go down . . . nine . . . eight . . . seven . . . six . . . five . . . four . . . three . . . two . . . one . . .

And now . . . now you are standing at the bottom of the set of stairs . . . and you walk forwards . . . into the cave . . . and hanging from the ceiling of the cave . . . on the walls . . . are hundreds of different varieties of minerals . . . There are red rubies . . . blue sapphires . . . and brilliant green emeralds . . . all of which are adorning the walls of the cave . . .

You can see the light as it plays and dances on the smoky citrine and sparkling amethyst . . . You can watch as light shines on the beautiful . . . subtle . . . colours of the rose quartz . . . You can feel . . . you can really feel the beautiful energy coming from this most wonderful of places . . . this most wonderful mineral kingdom . . .

Slight pause . . .

Looking deeper and deeper . . . deeper and deeper into the cave . . . , you notice a narrowing where the way in front . . . is lit with torches on the walls . . . You watch and marvel at the flames flickering against the backdrop . . . You begin to walk towards the light . . . until you see more steps . . . leading into the cave . . . deeper and deeper . . . deeper and deeper . . . and treading carefully now . . . Little pools of water are on the floor of the cave . . . small pools of water adorning the floor of the cave . . .

And now . . . now carefully you go down . . . deeper down . . . deeper and deeper down . . . to the deepest part of the cave . . . and as you do so . . . , the lights grow brighter as the cave widens and you come across a beautiful . . . magnificent . . . tropical garden . . .

A small path leads through to the garden . . . and on either side of the path are many and large . . . beautiful plants . . . You look around the garden again . . . and you can see small animals in the distance . . . There are huge ferns with bright and multicoloured foliage . . . There are deer and rabbits . . . There are squirrels . . . and you watch as a doe stops in her tracks . . . and stands on her hind legs . . . and turns . . . turns directly to look at you . . .

You stop and marvel at all the beauty of this place . . . and as you do so . . . , you begin to be aware . . . that the air is still and warm . . . humid . . . and on the trees are wonderful-looking butterflies . . . bigger and more brightly coloured than you ever thought was possible . . . You feel at one with both the plant and the animal kingdom . . . And once again you feel the radiant energy . . . from both the plants and the animals . . .

And now . . . now treading carefully . . . treading very carefully . . . along the stony path . . . you come to the end of this path . . . and it leads out . . . it leads out on to a small . . . beautiful . . . glistening bay . . . and in the bay, you can see the glistening bodies of the dolphins . . . playing . . . jumping . . . in the cool blue water . . .

The dolphins call for you . . . to join them . . . and you step down into the warm ocean . . . and they take you to their deepest secrets . . . and you swim along in their wake . . . and you feel at one with the dolphins . . . and all the creatures . . . the plants . . . that are in creation . . .

Long pause . . .

This is where you would do all your suggestion work . . .

And now . . now it is time to come back to the room . . . It is time to say goodbye to the dolphins . . . time to say goodbye to the plants . . . and the animals . . . It is time to say goodbye to the mineral kingdom . . . knowing that they are always there for you . . . They are always there for you . . .

Bring them slowly back . . .'

## Visualisation: Swimming

'I wonder now . . . if you can imagine that you are swimming in a large . . . and vast ocean . . . feel your body being supported in the water . . . feel the waves beneath you . . . splashing gently . . . as you move your arms . . . and your arms are moving . . . They are making the movements that you make for swimming . . . Imagine your arms as they push through the water . . . and as you do so . . . , your head is just above the waterline . . . with your legs . . . kicking and moving . . beneath you . . . You are swimming effortlessly . . . and moving calmly through the water . . .

And now . . . now in front of you . . . all that you can see . . . is the sea . . . and the vast ocean ahead of you . . . The sea goes on and on . . . on and on . . . for miles and miles . . . miles and miles . . . The sea is all around you . . . The sea is everywhere . . . and here in the sea . . . you are so small . . . in this enormous deep . . . blue . . . body of water . . . and as you effortlessly swim along . . . , you notice some splashes of water . . . as the fish dive out of the water . . . and back in again . . . all the time sending ripples alongside you . . . and the sea is a lovely shade of blue . . . going on . . . and on . . . and on . . . Imagine this scene now . . . Imagine yourself swimming in this vast ocean . . . safe and calm . . . calm and safe . . .

Pause for a short while . . .

And as you swim along . . . , your arms and your legs are moving . . . are moving in the movement of swimming . . . as you move through the water . . . easily . . . effortlessly . . . swimming along and going nowhere in particular . . . reaching no place in particular . . . just moving through the vast ocean . . . enjoying the peacefulness and serenity of this most wonderful of places . . .

Pause for a short while . . .

And now as you swim along . . . , you can see the horizon ahead of you . . . and over the horizon, the sun is just beginning to set . . . a glorious red and orange sunset . . . and you watch . . . you watch as you see the beautiful colours ahead of you . . . shades of red . . . changing from scarlet to a golden glow of orange . . . and spreading across the sea towards you . . . and as you watch sensational ripples of colour mingle with the pacific blue sea . . . which is becoming darker in shade . . . as you go further . . . further . . . further . . . and as it becomes darker in shade . . . , you begin to find that you can drift a little deeper . . . into those calm and tranquil feelings . . . that are now spreading throughout your entire body . . . and whilst you are swimming here . . . in this most wonderful places of yours . . . , think how nice it would be to rest . . . and completely let go . . . just completely rest . . . and totally relax and let go . . .

Pause for a short while . . .

And now . . . now the sun is going down right now . . . going down . . . over the sea . . . gradually diminishing . . . becoming a little smaller . . . as the reds and oranges . . . magically change to warmer shades of purple and violet . . . and the crimson darkening sky is streaked with golden yellow . . . in a breathtakingly . . . beautiful way . . .

Enjoy this view . . . Enjoy this wonderful view . . . and relax . . . relax a little deeper . . . just relax a little deeper now . . . letting go . . . letting go . . . and as the sun finally sets . . . , you find yourself drifting . . . drifting down to the bottom of the sea . . . You are still breathing . . . You are still breathing . . . deeply . . . evenly . . . and you listen to your breathing . . . slowly and rhythmically . . . breathing . . . and the sound of the waves in the ocean become one . . . as you nestle on the seabed . . . amongst the corals and reefs . . . and you look around you at the beautiful plant life . . . of the shoals of brightly coloured fish . . . that just swim on by . . .

And as you concentrate more and more on your breathing . . . , you begin to be aware that in a moment, I will be counting down from ten to zero . . . and with each number that I count . . . , you find that you can drift a little deeper . . . into calmness and comfort . . . You are safe and warm . . . warm and comfortable . . . here . . . here in your very own paradise . . .

Pause . . .

This is the part where you put your suggestions in for the benefit of the person you are working with . . .

Now . . . bring slowly and gently back . . .'

## Visualisation: Tropical Island

'Imagine that you are strolling along on a beautiful . . . tropical island . . . It is a warm and sunny afternoon . . . The sky is a lovely shade of blue . . . and the sea a startling shade of green and blue . . . The waves are dancing and splashing . . . up the shoreline . . . and the soft white sand is warm underneath your bare feet . . .

And . . . and as you begin to slowly walk further . . . further and further along . . . on the soft . . . white . . . sand . . . , you can feel the soft grains of sand beneath your toes . . . and as you take in this beautiful view . . . the beautiful blue-green sea . . . the lovely white sand . . . and the clear blue sky . . . , you feel calm and relaxed . . . relaxed and calm . . .

And now . . . now further along the beach . . . silhouetted against the blue sky . . . , there are palm trees . . . and chairs with shaded umbrellas . . . There is no one else around . . . but you . . . all you can hear and see are the sounds of the birds . . . singing somewhere in the distance . . . It is so calm here . . . It is so peaceful . . . This is your paradise . . . This is your very own paradise . . . your very own . . . private . . . place . . . where you can come and relax . . . at any time you wish . . . You can come here any time you want to . . . all within the power of your mind . . . All you need to do is relax . . . relax . . . relax . . .

And I wonder . . . I wonder if now . . . now you can imagine yourself sitting down here . . . finding a comfortable place to sit . . . on the soft . . . white sand . . . and as you find a comfortable place to sit . . . , you can see the sea . . . and the sparkling sunlight that reflects the ripples crossing the sea . . . Everything is calm . . . and so peaceful . . . and you can take into yourself . . . that calm and peaceful feeling . . . so calm . . . so peaceful . . . and so . . . so . . . tranquil . . .

You are just sitting there . . . on the soft white sand . . . and you can smell the fresh salt air . . . You can taste the fresh . . . salty . . . sea air . . . and you can taste it in your lungs . . . on your lips . . . so now . . . now experience that lovely fresh sea air . . . feel and experience that sea air . . . and as you breathe in pure air . . . deep into your lungs . . . , you experience that freshness and strength that it brings to you . . . Breathe in that lovely . . . fresh sea air . . . and just allow to see . . . how good it makes you feel . . . how good it does make you feel . . .

And as you are sitting there . . . just sitting there . . . listening to the sounds of the waves dancing and splashing against the shoreline . . . , you hear the sound of the seabirds in the distance . . . and as you do so . . . , you begin to feel a soft and gentle breeze against your skin . . . and the sun . . . so warm . . . against your body . . . You can feel the light from the sun radiating around your entire body . . . warming you gently . . . warming you so . . . so gently . . .

Just feel the warmth from the sun now . . . and imagine that you can direct the sunlight over your body . . . starting with both of your feet at the same time . . . Just begin to direct the warmth from the sun over both of your feet at the same time . . . and then up your legs . . . your calves . . . your shins . . . your thighs . . . your hips . . . your pelvic area and towards your stomach and chest . . . and now . . . now move the heat up and down your body . . . down and up . . . up and down . . . and then let it flow on over the shoulders and into the back . . . and all the way down the back of the body . . . and up again back to the shoulders and down the arms to the tip of the fingers . . .

Now . . . now move the heat up and down the arms . . . down and up . . . up and down . . . and then let it flow on up into the neck . . . the throat . . . and into the face . . . relaxing all of the facial muscles . . . and on up over the eyes and forehead into the crown of the head . . . Imagine the light from the heat of the sun entering the crown of the head and like a tornado soaring down the inside of the body . . . down and down . . . down and down . . . down . . . down . . .

Going deeper and deeper down . . . deeper and deeper down . . . and the further down you go, the more relaxed and more comfortable you become . . . calm and relaxed . . . relaxed and calm . . . until your entire body . . . from the top of your head . . . to the tips of your toes . . . are completely and totally relaxed . . . relaxed and calm . . . calm and relaxed . . .

And now . . . now I am going to count down from ten to one . . . and with each number . . . , I will take you deeper and deeper . . . deeper and deeper into total and complete relaxation . . . Ready now . . . ten . . . nine . . . eight . . . seven . . . six . . . five . . . four . . . three . . . two . . . one . . .'

This is where you will know enter the suggestions for the person that you are working with . . .

Now bring them slowly and gently back . . .

## Visualisation: Garden

'Now . . . now imagine that you are standing on a balcony overlooking a beautiful garden . . . It is a warm and beautiful summer's evening . . . and the air is filled with the fragrant smell of sweet scented flowers . . . Part of the garden is hidden from your view . . . and you really want to go behind there and look . . . to see what is hidden from your view . . . There are ten steps leading down . . . leading down from the balcony into the garden . . . and you begin to walk down the steps . . . counting with me in your mind . . . as you go down . . . Ready now . . .

Ten . . . nine . . . eight . . . seven . . . six . . . five . . . four . . . three . . . two . . . one . . .

And now . . . now you are standing at the bottom of the steps . . . and you can see in front of you . . . a small . . . grey . . . stony path . . . which winds itself through a wooden archway . . . and into the private garden . . . You can see clematis clinging to the archway . . . and next to the archway are weeping willows . . . looking magnificent in all their glory . . . Birds are singing tunefully in the trees . . . and there is a soft and gentle breeze . . . You can feel the air crossing your skin and on to your hair . . .

Walking through into the garden, you breathe in the scented night air . . . and feel the calmness it brings to you . . . It is so peaceful here . . . and it makes you feel calm . . . It makes you feel calm and relaxed . . . and you take . . . deep within yourself . . . that calm and relaxing feeling . . .

Experience this feeling now . . . feel that lovely . . . calm . . . relaxing feeling . . . It makes you feel so good . . . It makes you feel so relaxed . . . and you are becoming that calmer . . . more relaxed . . . And confident person . . . I want you to remember . . . to remember that you can relax like this anytime you wish . . . All you need to do . . . is to close your eyes for a moment . . . and think of the word *calm*.

Think of the word *calm* . . . and immediately you will feel just as calm . . . just as relaxed . . . as you do in your private garden . . .

Imagine now the word *calm* . . . Picture it written up there in your mind . . . on the screen of the mind . . . just inside the forehead . . . the word *calm* . . . or you could even hear the word being said in your mind . . . It might be my voice . . . Or it might be your voice . . . or it may be the voice of someone that you may . . . or may not . . . recognise . . .

You may even feel the word *calm* . . . in the centre of your very being . . . and this calmness is generated to every level of your being . . . and every cell in your body . . . receives the *calm* and peaceful feeling . . .'

This is where you would put the suggestions in for the person that you are working with . . .

Bring them back . . . slowly . . . gently . . . back . . .'

## Visualisation: Rose

*This is a very powerful induction that uses the imagination and the sense of smell—the oldest sense that we have. You will need to speak very slowly for the person to develop the images in his or her mind.*

'Imagine a beautiful golden light . . . entering through an opening in the crown of your head . . . and imagine the golden light . . . as it flows down through your face and into your neck . . . and your throat . . . Imagine it . . . Experience the energy from that golden light . . . and take it down . . . across the shoulders . . . down into the arms . . . and the hands . . . down into the chest . . . and focus that golden light around the heart area . . . and feel it gently pulsating . . . breathing . . . slowly . . . rhythmically . . .

Now . . . now down into the stomach . . . and feel and sense that wonderful feeling . . . the glowing . . . warming . . . sensation . . . melting . . . draining . . . down your body . . . into the hips . . . the thighs . . . the legs . . . the feet . . . and down to the toes . . .

And now . . . now the golden light enters your bloodstream . . . where . . . where it is then carried around the bloodstream . . . into the meridians . . . those little bursts of golden energy . . . and feel a sensation of peace . . . and letting go . . . letting go . . . letting go . . .

So now . . . now relax . . . and in your mind . . . imagine a beautiful red rose . . . in a tight round bud . . . The petals are as soft as velvet . . . and as you breathe in . . . , the rose very slowly begins to open . . . slowly opens . . . slowly unfolds . . . into a beautiful deep red rose . . . and with every breath, it opens more and more fully . . . into a lovely bloom . . . a beautiful deep red rose . . . rich and soft . . . and velvety . . . with a wonderful fragrance . . . like a rose garden on a warm summer's evening . . . and the perfume enters your nostrils . . . as it opens . . . fully . . . the petals spreading outwards . . . and you notice the centre of the rose . . . deep inside the rose . . . glowing . . . like a crimson sky aglow from a glorious sunset . . . and the glowing centre becomes brighter . . . a brighter shade of red . . . and the light begins to spread to the petals . . . until the whole rose is glowing with a bright . . . radiant . . . light . . .

And now . . . now with a sudden burst . . . the rose is a beautiful flame . . . and deep within . . . the shape of the rose . . . There is no heat . . . just pure energy combined with the beauty of the rose . . . The image is there . . . You can see it . . . You can sense the beauty of this wonderful flame . . . and the flame is confined . . . deep within the rose . . .

You can see it clearly in your mind's eye . . . and the energy vibrates . . . and you begin to breathe in that beautiful energy . . . It makes you feel so good . . . It makes you feel so relaxed . . . and it fills you completely with positive vibrations . . . higher vibrations . . . and just keep that image there in your mind . . . and focus on the rose as I continue to talk to your powerful subconscious mind . . . relax and let go . . . let go and relax . . .'

This is where you put the suggestions in for the person you are working with . . .

Bring back . . . bring slowly . . . gently back . . .'

## Visualisation: The Sunset

'And now . . . now in your imagination, I would like you to take yourself outside . . . to a beautiful place in nature . . . perhaps on a peaceful island . . . or maybe out in the country . . . This is your perfect setting . . . This is your very own special place . . .

Now . . . now I would like you to create a wonderful day . . . a warm . . . summer afternoon . . . or early evening . . . and a soft . . . gentle breeze caresses your skin and your hair . . . and there is nothing that you need to do right now . . . Just enjoy your very own special place . . .

Imagine yourself resting . . . maybe on a tree stump . . . or a cluster of rocks . . . watching your perfect scene . . . and the sun is beginning to set . . . as you watch as it gently lowers over the horizons . . . colouring the once blue sky . . . with beautiful splashes of colour . . . of crimson streaks . . . of yellow gold . . . that blends itself into the endless sky . . . as you sit and watch . . . as you just sit and watch . . .

And now . . . now before your eyes . . . the colours begin to change . . . begin to change as the sky becomes darker . . . purple colours drifting . . . lazily across the sky . . . and your mind begins to drift . . . begins to drift as you go deeper into hypnosis . . . deeper and deeper . . . deeper and deeper . . . as that most wonderful state of relaxation stays deep within you . . .

I would like you to enjoy this place . . . This is your very own special place . . . Allow the colours of the sunset fill your mind . . . and you may notice that the colours may change from time to time . . . Allow this to happen . . . as you watch the sun go down . . . as darkness begins to fall . . .

And now . . . now imagine a curtain . . . a veil . . . a cloak . . . or whatever your very own mind imagines . . . Being drawn across the sunset of your mind . . . the colours are still there and on the other side of the cloak, the colours are there also . . . but all that you see now . . . in your very own eyes is darkness . . . darkness in a place of colour . . . but is a comfortable place of darkness . . . It is safe . . . It is secure . . . It is like strong arms wrapped around a newborn child . . . that snuggles down into a comfortable and safe position . . . All its needs are met . . . both spiritually and physically . . .

You can now . . . now feel yourself drifting down . . . drifting down deeper and deeper . . . deeper and deeper . . . deeper within yourself . . . falling . . . descending . . . deeper and deeper relaxed . . . deeper and deeper relaxed . . .

And now . . . now allow yourself to think of an ocean . . . a beautiful blue ocean . . . and deep down . . . deep down on the ocean bed . . . another world exists . . . a world that you are not normally aware of . . . Allow yourself to feel part of this existence down here on the ocean bed . . . knowing that up there is the surface beneath the air . . . and the sky . . . and the world . . . You can marvel and see . . . the sun setting over the blue ocean . . .

It is a comfortable feeling down here . . . and there is a peaceful serenity deep within you . . . It makes you feel calm and relaxed . . . relaxed and calm . . . confident . . . calm . . . and relaxed . . .

This is the part where you put the suggestions in for the benefit of the person that you are working with . . .

Bring back . . . bring slowly . . . gently . . . back . . .'

## Hypnotherapy for Children

There are a few important differences between hypnotherapy with children and the techniques used and employed with adults. One of the most important differences is the use of vocabulary and the use of imagery; they should always be adapted and tailored to their developmental level, remembering that not all children can be assessed by their age alone.

- *Every child develops in their own way and in their own time and cannot be judged on age alone.*
- *When working with children, it is just as important to work with the parents and/or the carer, this will allow for a more successful outcome in the care plan.*
- *There is a more readier response and acceptance of the process.*
- *Children will often use self-hypnotic exercises more imaginatively and will experience pride in achieving the self-mastery (often allowing for the natural self—healing to take place)*
- *It is generally agreed that hypnotic techniques in any formal sense cannot be used with children below the age of four.*
- *You do not have to use a progressive relaxation with children.*

I have included some hypnotherapy scripts for you to use; they can either be used as they are or adapted to suit the child's needs. Remember, imagination is the key, and they are more likely to accept the suggestions that you make, allowing the story to flow, and the use of metaphors is of great benefit.

**Football visualisation for children (you can adapt football to other sports that are of interest, and for more impact, use the child's name)**

'Picture yourself at a football match . . . You have the best seat in the stadium, and it gives you a perfect view of the football pitch . . . and all the players down there . . . You are wearing the colours of the team that you support . . . It is cold . . . but not too cold . . . and you are comfortably wrapped up . . . with layers and layers of clothing . . .

Notice who you are with . . . a friend . . . a parent . . . or maybe even a crowd of others . . . See your favourite player . . . (name the player here) . . . about to kick the football . . . and the opposition are trying to get in there first . . . but . . . (name the player here) . . . is too quick . . . and he has kicked the ball . . . It is going up in the air now . . . across the pitch . . . and towards the net . . . Everyone is shouting . . . and cheering . . . and the goalkeeper tries to stop the ball from entering the net, but it is too late . . . The ball has crossed the line . . . It is a goal . . .

The other players run up to him . . . and hug him . . . and the crowd are cheering . . . There is a wonderful atmosphere here . . . It is exciting . . . It is exhilarating . . . You love the feeling of being here . . . of watching this game of football . . .

You are jumping up and down . . . You feel so good . . . You feel so good . . .

Stop . . . You notice . . . (name of your hero here) . . . Look . . . he is looking up at you . . . and your eyes meet . . . and he winks at you . . . He is sharing with you a special moment . . . and as your eyes become locked with his . . . for just a fraction of a second . . . and yet . . . yet it seems to last for hours . . . You feel inside of you . . . you feel inside that you have a wonderful feeling of accomplishment . . . of achievement . . .

Now . . . now I would like you to change the scene down there . . . It is you down there . . . and you are running across the football pitch . . . You are wearing shorts . . . and a t-shirt . . . and you are wearing boots . . . and you feel the boots on the ground . . . It is hard beneath your feet . . . and you are running towards the ball . . .

Now . . . now run the scene again . . . but this time, it is you that scores the goal . . . You are concentrating on the ball . . . You mind is focused and alert . . . and you single-mindedly go towards the goal . . . You are a success . . . You are a winner . . . and it is a wonderful . . . tremendous feeling . . . and as the ball goes into the net . . . , you feel so good . . . that you could jump high into the air . . . You have scored . . . You have succeeded . . . You have done it . . . You hear the crowd cheering and clapping their hands . . . shouting your name . . . and the other players hugging you . . . making you feel good . . . making you feel so very good . . .

You now focus . . . you now focus entirely on that feeling of success . . . and you make those good feelings grow stronger . . . You feel confident . . . You feel positive . . . You know that you are a success . . . and you can achieve whatever you have set out to achieve . . . You enjoy feeling this way . . . and it is a feeling that you are getting used to . . . and because you focus your mind on success . . . , this success spreads to all areas of your body . . . to all areas of your body . . .'

This is the part where you put the suggestions in for the child you are treating . . .

Now bring back . . . slowly . . . gently . . . back . . .'

## Relaxation for Children (speak very slowly and in a softer tone)

'Would you like to play a new game with me called Let's Pretend? . . . You would . . . That's great . . .

OK . . . this is what we do . . . I am going to tell you a story . . . and I want you to close your eyes . . . and pretend as hard as you can . . . that you can see all the things that are in this story . . . Are you OK with that? . . . That's good . . . That's very good . . .

First of all, I would like you to wonder . . . to wonder if you can pretend if you can be a big . . . rag . . . doll . . . Do you know . . . do you know that rag dolls are soft and floppy . . . ? See if you can make your very own arm . . . your very own right arm . . . floppy . . . and tell me when you think it is . . .

Wait for response . . .

Good . . . very good . . . Let's test that then, shall we? . . . I will lift up your right hand and let it drop gently on to the bed (you can use a chair, your lap, or whatever feels right for both of you) . . . and if your hand is really . . . really . . .

floppy . . . , then your right hand will drop down . . . will drop down . . . all floppy . . .

(*This is where you lift up the child's hand and drop it gently. If the child's hand goes down slowly, then they are not fully relaxed. You can demonstrate how you want them to do this. Arm hand needs to go down quickly for them to be relaxed enough.*)

Now . . . now see if you can close your eyes . . . and just pretend that the eyelids are stuck together . . . , pretend that they are stuck so tightly together that the eyelids will not open at all . . .

(*If the child opens his or her eyes, then you can tell them that they are not pretending hard enough, and you can repeat the request again; however, some children insist on keeping their eyes open all the way through. Do not worry. They can still visualise well with their eyes open.*)

I want you to imagine that you are a young bird . . . and that you have just learned to fly . . . on your own . . . on your very own . . . You have been out with your mummy and daddy . . . a few times now . . . and now is the time . . . Now is the time for you to go on an adventure . . . an adventure about you flying up into a lovely blue sky . . .

Your very own wings are flapping up and down . . . as your body lifts up higher and higher . . . higher . . . and higher . . . and higher . . . and the higher up that you go . . . , the smaller everything below you look . . . and the more comfortable that you feel . . . and when you are as high as you would like to go . . . I would like you to slow down a little . . . slow down and take a look at the earth beneath you . . .

And as you look down . . . , you can see that you are flying over a field of lovely . . . bright . . . yellow flowers . . . and around the edge of the field . . . , there is a row of trees . . . and on the other side of the row of trees is a pretty-looking stream . . . and now . . . now because you are a bird . . . flying up high in the sky . . . , you have a very special eyesight . . . and you can see right down into that stream . . . and you can see some tiny fish . . . swimming around . . . around some smooth round pebbles . . . and swimming around also . . . are some tiny black tadpoles . . . darting here and there . . . growing out of the stream are some long . . . long . . . blades of green grass . . . and you notice a few white lily leaves . . . Sitting on one of the lily leaves is a green frog . . .

You look around to see what else you can see . . . You may see a rabbit peeping out from behind one of those trees . . . or perhaps a grasshopper . . . or a ladybird . . . What colour is the ladybird? . . . How many spots does she have? . . . Across the field is an ant . . . scuttling across the grass . . . and he is carrying something on his back . . .

And as you look down . . . as you look down on all those creatures . . . , you become very curious about what it is they are doing . . . and you begin to fly down . . . You begin to fly down to join them . . . and you feel yourself going down . . . going down . . . down . . . down . . .

And as your feet touch the floor . . . , an amazing thing begins to happen . . . You are back to yourself again . . . a little boy called (name of boy here) . . . who is three years old . . . and the ladybird has changed into (name a little girl that lives next door or in the bed next to them in the hospital) . . . and the rabbit has changed into (name some friends here or a nurse) . . . and all your friends are here . . . with you . . .

And today . . . this moment in time . . . you are all going to go on a magic journey . . . and, suddenly, everything around you is changing . . . is changing into a wonderful . . . magic . . . playground . . . and you see a magic roundabout that goes round and round . . . round and round . . . round and around . . . and around . . . and around . . . and around . . . I can only wonder what you will feel like when you get off this roundabout . . .

Next . . . next you begin to wobble over to me . . . to the swings . . . and you now sit on one of those swings . . . The seat is hard beneath your bottom . . . and you can feel your fingers . . . around the cold metal chain . . . and you push your feet back . . . and then out . . . to make yourself go higher . . . higher and higher . . . higher and higher . . . and higher . . . higher . . . higher . . . up . . . up . . . up . . . until you can see for miles and miles around . . .

Soon the swing . . . begins to slow down . . . and, eventually, it stops . . . and you jump off easily . . . and run over to the slide . . . and from the top of the slide, you glide easily and smoothly down . . . You go down and down . . . down and down . . . down . . . down . . . down . . .

And whilst you are drifting deeper and deeper down . . . , you can begin to wonder about what you will see at the bottom of this slide . . . There could be elves . . . fairies . . . princes and kings . . . There could even be wizards or magicians . . . I can only wonder what it is that you will discover at the bottom of this slide . . .

And when you reach the bottom of this slide . . . , you can go and join your new friends for a wonderful adventure . . . You can drift into dreamland . . . You can swim oceans . . . or fly into space . . . You can do anything that you want . . . because you can . . . because it is a magical . . . mystical . . . place . . . it is your very own special place . . .

And . . . and because you are in your very own special place . . .

This is where you can put the suggestions in for the person that you are working with . . .

And now . . . now I want you to know that you can come back here anytime that you wish . . . and that this is your very own special place . . . your very own special place . . .

Bring back . . . bring slowly . . . gently back . . .

***Children have wonderful imaginations, and the following three inductions can be used to suit the particular child in question.***

## The Secret Place

'Close your eyes . . . and imagine being somewhere that is really nice . . . maybe someplace you have been on holiday . . . or someplace with your friends . . . I can really bet that you can imagine this scene so well . . . It feels as if you are really there . . .

And you know . . . you know what it is like when you think of something that is pleasant and exciting . . . You can feel really good . . . right now . . . right now in this moment of time . . . This is your very own special place . . . your secret place . . . It can be a magic place . . . where anything you want to happen . . . can happen . . . You can give it a name if you would like . . . a special name . . . a secret name . . .

And . . . and you do not have to tell me where your very own special place is . . . or even what that secret name is . . . because this place . . . and this name . . . belongs to you . . . and you alone . . . and . . . and because anytime you want to feel better . . . You can always go . . . You can always go into your imagination . . . to your safe and secret place . . . All you have to do is say the name to yourself . . . It is like your very own secret password . . . and when you do . . . , you can imagine being there . . . really safe . . . really . . . really . . . safe . . .'

You can now use the suggestions that you want to use . . .

Bring back . . . slowly . . . gently . . . back . . .

# The Magic TV

*Ask the child to close their eyes until you tell them to open them, ask them about their favourite TV programme, then when he has finished telling you, as those about the part of the TV programme that he enjoys most of all.*

*Continue with the following words:*

'And now . . . now . . . in a moment . . . with your eyes closed . . . you will begin seeing your very own favourite TV programme . . . You will feel calm and relaxed . . . relaxed and calm . . . You will feel peaceful and safe . . . safe and peaceful . . . Now . . . now I am turning on the TV right now . . . and in your mind, you will see your favourite programme on the screen . . .

And . . . and on that screen . . . you will hear the sounds . . . and have the feelings of enjoying and watching . . . your very own favourite programme . . . You can continue to watch that TV programme by keeping your eyes closed . . . and you do not have to listen to what it is that I am saying . . . You just continue to relax and enjoy that special programme . . . by keeping your eyes closed . . . until I tell you to open them and wake up . . .

Now . . . now in a moment . . . that programme will finish . . . and we will change the channel . . . and you will continue to move into an even deeper state . . . You will be seeing a programme that . . . that will . . .'

This is the part where you would put the suggestions in for the benefit of the child you are working with . . .

Bring back . . . slowly . . . safely . . . back . . .

## The Flying Blanket

'Imagine that you are going on a picnic . . . going with your very favourite people . . . to a special place . . . for a picnic . . . You have all your favourite things to eat and drink . . . you can see . . . and you can smell them . . . you can even taste them . . .

And as you imagine that food . . . , I want you to enjoy playing games with your family and friends . . . enjoy all the games that you like to be playing . . . and when you are tired . . . and when you cannot play any games anymore . . . and when you cannot eat or drink . . . any of that lovely food anymore . . . i want you to sit down . . .

Not to sit down just anywhere . . . but to sit down on a special blanket . . . and this blanket is made of your very favourite colour . . . you see that blanket spread all over the ground . . . made of your very own favourite colour . . . and that colour is . . . (insert favourite colour) . . . smooth and soft . . . soft and smooth is this blanket . . . and you may . . . when you wish to . . . sit on this blanket . . . You may even would like to lie on this blanket . . . You could even pretend that this is a very special flying blanket . . .

And this very special flying blanket . . . allows you even to be a pilot . . . You and the blanket can fly together . . . You are the pilot . . . and you are in control . . . You can fly this blanket . . . just a few inches above the ground . . . just above the grass below you . . . or if you want . . . , you can even fly this blanket higher above the trees if you want to . . . always in control . . . always feeling safe . . . safe and in control . . . in control and safe . . .

You are the pilot . . . and you can go where you want to . . . and as fast . . . or as slow as you wish . . . all by just thinking about it . . . in your mind . . . imagining it in your very own mind . . .

And do you know . . . do you know that you can land . . . You can land and visit your friends . . . You can land at the zoo . . . You can land anywhere that you would like . . . You are the pilot . . . and you are in control . . . You are in charge . . .

You might even fly by a tree . . . and see birds in a nest . . . You can speed up and slow down . . . You can enjoy wherever it is you would like to go . . . Take all the time you need to feel very comfortable . . . and when you are ready . . .

when you are ready, you can find a nice . . . comfortable . . . safe . . . landing spot . . . to rest comfortably yourself . . . and your flying blanket . . . and when you have landed . . . , you can let me know by lifting one of your fingers of your hand . . .'

Now is the time you can put in the suggestions for the child that you are working with . . .

Bring slowly . . . gently . . . back . . .

# STRENGTH AND COURAGE

As I come to the end of this book, I would like to leave you with just a few thoughts. As we go through the journey of life, it takes us on many, many paths. It is up to us which path we choose and whatever path you have decided to walk down; remember that it is undeniably the right one.

We meet many people along the way, and it is with an open heart that I thank you for reading this book, and I hope and pray that you have the strength, courage, and wisdom to carry on walking the path on your journey, not only in this lifetime but also in others to come.

Remember, we and we alone have the power within us to heal our mind and our body, and with this in mind, I offer you the following script so that you may use to have the strength, courage, and wisdom to heal your very own mind . . . and . . . body.

With love and honour

Carl

AHO

'And as you continue now . . . drifting deeper and deeper with every outward breathe that you take . . . I would like you to imagine yourself in a beautiful garden . . . a place of tranquillity and peace . . . and here you are safe and secure . . . and all around you is nature's beauty and colours . . . There are flowers and shrubs . . . tall trees that provide cooling shade from the rays of the sun that are filtering down through the leaves . . . and the branches of the magnificent ancient trees . . .

A little way off... ahead of you... is an archway... covered with sweet-smelling honeysuckle... and there is a wonderful water feature... and the water is sparkling in the sunlight... as it cascades over the rocks... and into a large pool below... that is filled with water lilies... There are fish swimming in this pool... and you watch in wonder... as one of those fish breaks the surface to feed... and you find it so easy to relax here... to let go completely of cares and concerns... and drifting with those thoughts... that allow for change... as you and the world around changes... all around you...

And... and as you continue to relax here... lying on a carpet of lush green lawn... the grass is cool against your skin... and you recognise now... you recognise that this is really a wonderful... special... place... a healing place... a place where so many have come before you... have come to enjoy the peace and harmony... the peace and harmony of the healing powers of the holy men and women... those who have arrived here throughout the ages... sent here by an almighty power to attend to those who have suffered... and I want you now to relax... to relax... and continue to drift and dream... as you wait for your very own healer to come...

Pause for one minute...

That's good... That's very good... You are doing so really well... and now... now I wonder if you can hear a voice calling you... calling your name... and the sound comes nearer and nearer... nearer and nearer... soothing... calming... healing... this is your healer... This is your very own special healer... moving closer to you now... moving closer and closer... closer and closer... and closer... now...

And as your healer moves closer to you..., a creature of pure light... a person of wisdom... a person of infinite wisdom... is sent to you... from the very power that transcends all... and you feel that power now... a gentle power... a gentle warming sensation... that flows through your body... and you feel that power now... spreading from the top of your head... and as your healer touches you there... a growing sense of well-being... begins to move through every cell in your body... every muscle... every fibre of your being... calming... calming... calming your mind...

And as your mind begins to calm... you realise your healer has brought you a gift... a gift of strength... of courage... a gift that may be with you as you face your journey ahead... At all times... that will never leave your side... a true gift of strength... courage... and wisdom...

You have standing by your side . . . your very own healer . . . and standing next to your healer is a tiger . . . not just any tiger . . . but a tiger that will be there for you on your journey ahead . . . and no harm will come to you from this tiger . . . this tiger is here for your protection . . . for your guide . . . as you walk your path ahead . . .

So now . . . now the tiger introduces themselves to you . . . and they tell you their name . . . there very special name . . . that you . . . and you alone . . . will be able to call them by . . . and whenever you need to call your tiger . . . All you have to do is call their name . . . their very own special name . . . and the tiger will be there with you . . . standing by your side . . . your very own special tiger . . . your very own special healer . . . right by your side . . .

And now . . . now as your special healer works on you . . . you can feel that healing more and more . . . more and more now . . . stimulating your own natural healing forces . . . and those healing forces from within . . . do their very best for you now . . . seeking out those discomforts . . . soothing and relaxing . . . encouraging blood flow . . . encouraging vital blood flow which carries around the vital oxygen . . . the vital nutrients . . . through your whole body . . . and every organ is richly nourished . . . your very own body's defence system moving . . . and seeking out all intrusions . . . regenerating . . . stimulating . . . purifying . . . and healing . . . and as your healer continues . . . moving hands . . . healing hands . . . over your body . . . concentrating on those parts that need the most attention . . . spreading warmth . . . that glowing sensation . . . of oneness . . . with the universe . . . a growing sensation that spreads . . . and cocoons you . . . surrounding you entirely in healing light . . . as you hear the words deep within . . . deep within your inner mind . . . and as your own personal and wise higher self . . . absorbs that concentration of positive power . . . it increases your feelings of self-worth . . . of confidence . . . relaxing you in this very special way . . .

And now . . . and now as your healer fades away into the distance . . . , your very own tiger is standing next to you . . . standing next to you . . . giving you strength and courage in your journey ahead . . . to push back the barriers in your life . . . to push back the barriers as you walk with each and every step . . . pushing back the barriers . . . you and your tiger . . . with each . . . and every . . . step . . . pushing back the barriers . . . pushing back the barriers . . .'

Carl has produced the following CD titles to accompany his book, which are also available in MP3 format. Each CD has been produced in a recording studio using state-of-the-art equipment and sound. Carl has used the very latest hypnotherapy techniques to enhance relaxation, enabling the absorption of powerful suggestions, in a caring and safe way.

- Your Very Own Special Place
- Loss of a Loved One
- Dying Regrets: The Top Five Regrets of the Dying
- The Dying Process: A Transition From Life to Death
- Living With Cancer: Relaxation for Chemotherapy
- Living With Cancer: Relaxation for Fighting Cancer
- Living With Cancer : Fear of Needles and Fear of Blood
- Visualisations 1 Dolphin Experience and Swimming in the Sea
- Visualisations 2 Tropical Island and the Sunset
- Visualisations for Children 1 Football Visualisation and The Flying Blanket(With Free Bonus Induction Track )

All CDs are priced at £11.95 each and MP3 at £10.95 each

Postage and packing will be applied at the current rate (price available on request).

In producing these cds Carl has used the latest in sound, with 528hz sound effects which enable for complete relaxation. 528hz is a simple mathematical number that is central to the "musical matrix of creation", this "love vibration" resonates in your heart connecting you to the reality of heaven and earth," a oneness with the source of creation.

# Contact Details

Carl gathern

Mid Sussex Therapies

Ivy House

Henfield High Street

Henfield

West Sussex

Bn5 9hn

United Kingdom

carlgathern@gmail. com

www. midsussextherapies. co. uk

# Coming Soon

The next book Carl is writing is *Stress and Anxiety? Would You Like More Confidence? Hypnotherapy Can Help*

# Chapter 1

## Stress Management

The human brain receives messages from several sources, each dealing with separate types of information (this is both internal and external).

The conscious mind deals with reasoning and logic, decisions, goal planning, and all conscious activity.

The unconscious mind receives all the messages from our social, spiritual, and genetic backgrounds and all the conflicts and disturbances which enter our subconscious each day.

The unconscious mind receives and holds its information, neither accepting nor rejecting the messages; it does not evaluate, leaving it to the conscious mind.

From primitive times, the human mind has possessed an escape mechanism that even today, under severely threatening conditions, can cause regression to primitive behaviour.

The fight or flight syndrome, always a mean of dealing with fears, threat attacks, and other disturbances, has gained tolerance through evolution.

The desire for social acceptance provides us with the motivation to cope with and adapt with reality.

>We can't fight the environment, so *what now?*

## Enter Stress and Anxiety

Unable to fight, reaction turns to flight, which in present life can prove impossible.

Often a state of apathy, depression and/or hyper-suggestibility happens. Negative input finds acceptance, and an overreaction to the senses develops with a loss of tolerance, which, in turn, leads to a downward spiral.

A person who is experiencing such symptoms may well suffer with stress and anxiety.

Certain types of stress are desirable, such as job promotions, but stresses that are producing debilitation, depression, anger, grief, over-eating, and similar reactions needs attention.

The first recognition of a therapist dealing with stress is likely to be that while the world. Or the past, if it is a factor in the condition, cannot be changed, it is possible to alter the clients perception of and the reaction to them.

Stress may be a reaction to people, places, events, situations, and the threats may be real or imagined. The subconscious mind does not analyse, and usually by the time depression appears, the conscious mind has lost the ability to do so.

There are several common causes of stress, which can be defined and eliminated.

## What's behind it all?

Why me? Stress victims ask the question quite often, and many factors enter into the realm of possibilities. They can also be addicted to stress, enjoy it, until it get's out of control.

Victims can learn stress early in life from experiences, which they consider a normal part of everyday life.

Fears, valid or not, can lead to the onset of stress, which can then expand into phobias.

Repressed emotions, such as hurt, anger, and grief, are a very worrying, concerned over health, while certain medical conditions, including dietary deficiencies, can lead to stress and PMS.

Every individual is different in tolerance levels, coping abilities, and reactions, and their therapeutic needs and dealing with stress is best accomplished by a trained, experienced, and sensitive professional, who can determine the cause.

The effectiveness and desensitisation can be brought about by hypnotherapy, using counselling and NLP skills.

Through the process of hypnotherapy, positive new responses can be created to replace the devastating response of the past.

Buried feelings can be brought to the surface and released. Outside pressure can be relieved, and, finally, new responses to old disturbances can be included, with major changes in both attitudes and reactions.

Want to know more? Then read on . . .

# Index

## A

acceptance  42-3, 53, 66, 71-2, 98, 161, 178
acute pain  93, 96-7, 100
adults  17, 19, 42, 161
age  17, 25, 48, 149, 161, 171
air  84-5, 101, 150, 152, 156-7, 161-3
American Institute of Hypnosis  29
anaesthesia  13-14, 27-8, 82, 92, 98, 102, 108, 149-50
analgesics  91
anger  15, 47, 53, 55, 66, 71-2, 178-9
animal magnetism  26
ankles  57
anti-bodies  80
anxiety  15, 17, 38, 50, 52-3, 55, 93-4, 96-7, 100, 105, 107, 175, 178
archway  157, 171
arms  36, 41, 57, 66, 68, 106-7, 121, 127-9, 142-3, 153-4, 156, 158, 163
attention  26-8, 31-2, 35-6, 44, 46, 54, 79, 88, 178
awareness  32-3, 35, 54, 107, 135

## B

barriers  111, 172
battle  76, 88-9
bed  41, 68, 150, 163, 165
behaviours  30, 33, 111-12, 116, 124
belief system  73, 105, 114
beta waves  34
blood  19-20, 146-9, 173
  fear of  146, 148-9, 173
body  12, 18-23, 33-4, 39-40, 51, 66-8, 75-7, 82-9, 91-9, 102-3, 124-5, 127-8, 156, 163-4, 170-2
body temperature  40, 68
bone marrow  19-20
bones  19-20
brain  30, 34, 37, 52, 79-80, 92-5, 97, 99, 114-16
brain waves  34, 84
breasts  18-19
breathing  23, 33, 35, 41, 56, 68, 84, 106-8, 114, 118-20, 124, 154-5, 158
British Medical Association  28-9
British Society of Clinical and Experimental Hypnosis  32

## C

calmness  35, 84, 129, 155, 157-8, 171
cancer  5, 11-14, 16-22, 38-9, 46-8, 50-1, 55, 74-6, 86, 91-2, 97, 100, 112, 138, 173
  brain  20
  breast  17
  common types of  17, 19
  diagnosis of  39, 41
  lung  7, 12, 17
  prostate  17
  rectal  17
cancer patients  11, 16, 51, 55
cancer treatments  13, 20, 47, 50
carcinomas  19
carers  11, 16, 38, 41, 68, 161
cells  18-20, 75, 83-4, 86-90, 158, 171
  blood  19-20
  cancer  12-13, 75-7, 80
  cancerous  80, 89
  connective tissue  19-20
  epithelial  19
  healthy  80, 88-9
  malignant  87, 89-90
  nerve  93-5
chemotherapy  5, 12-13, 20-1, 48, 51, 75, 77, 173
chest  57, 119-20, 127, 156, 158
clients  13, 21, 28-9, 91, 98, 111-12, 122
colon  17-18
comfort  45-6, 81, 102, 155
conscious critical faculty (CCF)  105-6, 108-9, 131
consciousness  25-6, 33-6, 83, 105, 108-9, 123, 138
courage  5, 44-5, 61-2, 140, 170-2
curative treatments  48

## D

daydreaming  31, 35, 37
death  5, 11, 22-4, 38-42, 60-1, 65-9, 92, 149, 173
deep hypnosis  35-6, 144, 150
depression  13, 15, 43, 53, 66, 71, 178
diagnosis  12, 50-1, 53, 55, 74, 97
discomfort  51-2, 80, 82, 95, 102, 128, 141, 147, 172
discovery  27-9, 39, 66, 83, 92
disease  21-2, 26, 48, 51, 55, 74, 80, 84, 91, 93, 97
distance  85, 133, 148, 152, 155-6, 172
doctors  11, 14, 16, 18, 75, 82, 85, 96-7, 141, 143-6
dreams  15, 44, 61-2, 83-4, 171
driving  31-2

## E

electrical activity  34
emotional experience  91, 139
emotional issues  14
emotions  15, 33, 38, 43, 45, 47, 53, 65, 72-3, 95-6, 112, 117, 120, 129
empathy  112
endorphins  94-5, 99
energy  22, 29, 40, 67-8, 83, 85, 158-9
Erickson, Milton H.  29-30
Esdaile, James  27, 108
experience  12-13, 16, 32, 37, 42-3, 52, 95-6, 104-6, 115-16, 123-4, 126, 139-40, 144-5, 147-8, 156-8
  past  35, 42, 96, 139, 141
eyelids  107, 127, 164
eyes  12, 22-3, 35-6, 41, 56-7, 59, 68, 107-8, 121-4, 127-9, 135, 144-5, 160, 162-4, 166-7

## F

family  15-16, 23, 38, 42-3, 48-50, 53, 97, 168
fear  13, 15-16, 34, 45, 47, 50-1, 63, 66, 68, 96, 98, 138-48, 177-8
feelings  15, 36, 50-4, 58-60, 62, 72, 83-4, 95, 106-7, 112-13, 115-17, 138, 142, 148-51, 162-3
focus  13-14, 16, 33, 53, 84, 109, 112-13, 115, 120, 127-31, 134, 158-9, 163
food  40-1, 67-8, 84, 168
free association  28, 33-4

## G

garden  101, 150, 152, 157-9
goals  14-15, 46, 48-9, 109, 162
grief  12, 38, 41-3, 70-1, 178-9
gustatory  120-1

## H

hair loss  77
harmony  83, 90, 119, 133, 171
head  22, 57, 80, 120, 124, 127, 129, 135, 153, 156, 158, 171
healer  171-2
healing  14, 28, 33, 35, 50, 53, 77, 80, 82, 84, 96, 102-3, 109, 124-6, 171-2
health  44, 62, 84-5, 179
hearing  14, 23, 41, 68, 113, 116, 119, 147
heart  73, 87, 97, 145-6
home  23, 47, 54, 81
hospice  22, 38, 46, 53, 55, 92, 100, 110, 112, 138
hospital  14, 47, 51, 165
hot flushes  13
hypnosis  5, 11, 13, 25-37, 43, 50-2, 54-5, 79, 93-4, 97-8, 105-9, 114, 125-6, 129-30, 149-50
hypnotherapist  11-12, 21, 32, 91, 99, 108, 139
Hypnotherapy  11-17, 21-7, 29-30, 32-3, 37-9, 41, 45-7, 49-55, 91-3, 95-7, 99-101, 107, 149-51, 161, 179

## I

illnesses  16, 45, 48-9, 52-3, 62, 80, 86, 92, 94, 96
images  79, 99, 123, 132, 137, 144, 158-9
imagination  52, 76, 83, 86, 118, 122, 125, 131, 151, 158-9, 161, 167
immune system  12-13, 51, 54, 80
induction  32, 116, 125-6, 129, 131, 158, 166
information  30, 52, 104-5, 110, 112-13, 116, 121, 177
initial consultation  110-11, 124
internal dialogue  121-2

## K

kinaesthetic  117, 122

## L

lateral eye movements (LEM)  121
legs  36, 41, 57, 68, 106-7, 153-4, 156, 158
leukaemia  17, 20
life  5, 16, 21-2, 24, 31-2, 38-40, 43-50, 53, 61, 63-8, 73, 79, 83-7, 97-8, 144-5
loss  5, 12, 15, 35, 38, 41-3, 51, 70-2, 107, 173, 178

love  9, 16, 38, 70, 72-3, 85, 142, 144, 162, 170
lymphatic system  19-20
lymphomas  20

## M

medical profession  15, 21, 26, 145-6
medicine  28-9, 76, 94, 149
melanoma  17
memories  67, 73, 79, 86, 107, 144
Mesmer, Dr.  26-7
mesmerism  27
mind  12-13, 33-4, 57-8, 79, 82-5, 96-8, 104-5, 110-11, 123-4, 127-8, 130-2, 143-51, 157-60, 167-8, 170-1
  conscious  14, 31-5, 104-5, 131, 177-8
  subconscious  32-6, 50, 60, 79, 82, 86, 90, 104-5, 109, 123, 131, 144, 146, 149, 159
  unconscious  14, 33, 177
mobility  15, 92
modalities  115-21
morphine  94
mortality  39
movements  40, 68, 104, 120, 153-4
muscles  19, 36, 57, 86, 124-5, 127, 137, 171

## N

nausea  13, 33, 47-8, 51-2, 138
needles  52, 82, 140-3, 173
  fear of  138-9, 142, 148, 173
neurolinguistic programming (NLP)  29-30, 179
nurses  11, 22, 43, 61, 75, 82, 85, 143, 165

## O

olfactory  120
operation  14, 27, 82-3, 97, 143-5, 149-51

## P

pain  12, 27, 46, 48-9, 51-2, 55, 86, 91-100, 107-8, 128, 137, 151
  control of  91, 97-9
  perception of  92, 95, 98-9
painkillers  94-5, 97
palliative care  22, 38, 44, 46-9, 53-5, 61, 92, 100, 110, 112, 138
panic  139
patients  11, 16, 21-2, 26-7, 32, 38-9, 42, 44, 47-55, 61, 82, 91-2, 98-100, 104, 146
peace  11, 23, 45-6, 55, 59, 62, 69-72, 83-4, 97, 107, 133, 142-3, 151, 159, 170-1
phobias  33, 51, 138-41, 147-8, 178
physical body  36, 52, 92
postures  111, 113, 118-20
power  50, 97, 99-100, 110, 123, 125, 150, 155, 170-1
problems  21, 48, 60, 80, 94, 145, 149
process  16, 39, 43, 53-4, 66-7, 92-5, 100, 121-2, 126-8, 161, 179
psychoanalysis  28
psychotherapy  26, 30, 33

## R

rapport  110-11, 113
receptors  93-5
regrets  40, 44, 53, 61-3, 67, 69, 173
relaxation  5, 12, 33-4, 52, 54, 56, 60, 75, 79, 81, 84, 86, 106-8, 135, 173
relief  48-9, 55, 76, 91-2, 94, 96, 100, 107
reorganisation  42-3
reorientation  125-6, 138
representations  37, 116
resolution  28, 42-3
response  94, 111, 137, 163, 179

## S

sarcomas  20
science  32, 34, 39, 92, 94
scripts  55-6, 60, 65, 70, 75, 79, 82, 86, 98, 100, 104, 107, 109, 116-17, 121-5
  authoritarian  122-3, 125
  permissive  122-3, 125
self-hypnosis  12-14, 32, 52, 54, 75, 103
sensations  36-7, 52, 76, 92, 95, 148, 158-9, 171
senses  35, 37, 52, 110, 115-16, 121, 123, 178
signals  88-9, 93, 99, 128
skin  18-19, 87, 102, 141, 156-7, 160, 171
sleep  27, 36, 40, 67, 107, 115, 134
smell  78, 94, 120, 123, 148, 156, 158, 168
special place  58-60, 65, 70, 75, 77-8, 80, 82-3, 85, 123, 125-6, 135-8, 141-2, 150, 160, 166
speech  68, 111, 118-19, 121
spinal cord  92-3
stress  12, 17, 48, 50-1, 91, 96, 98, 138, 175, 178-9
success  26, 50, 104-5, 108, 120, 125, 162-3
suggestion work  99, 107-10, 125-6, 129, 136, 153
sun  83, 99, 133, 154, 156, 160, 170
surgeons  14, 27, 75, 82, 145-6, 149-50
surgery  13, 20-1, 27, 38, 51, 83, 85, 91, 97, 108, 149-50
survival instincts  105

## T

techniques  13, 27, 29, 52, 109, 126, 139, 161
therapies  20-1, 25, 32, 49, 108-9
therapist  29, 32, 107, 178
theta waves  35
trance  12, 25-7, 31-3, 35-6, 79, 87, 105-7, 129-31, 135, 137-8
treatment  12-13, 18, 20-1, 47-9, 53-5, 74-5, 77, 80, 93, 96-7, 99-100, 110, 138, 146

## V

visualisations  151, 153, 155, 157-9, 173
voice  56, 58, 60, 64-5, 73, 78-9, 83, 88, 111, 113-14, 118-19, 124, 126, 137, 158

## W

Ware, Bronnie  44
warmth  76, 80-1, 83, 143, 156
well-being  50, 81, 85, 138, 140, 143, 149, 171
white light  80-1
wisdom  44, 61, 170-1
women  17, 44, 62, 94, 171
worries  17, 23, 50, 75, 77, 83, 105, 126, 145, 164